M000105591

# Scripture Yoga:

## 21 Bible Lessons
## for Christian Yoga Classes

*Susan Neal RN, MBA, MHS*

Please consult with a healthcare professional before performing yoga postures or any new type of exercise program. If you have a special medical condition, you should consult with your doctor regarding possibly modifying the program contained in this book. The author assumes no responsibility for any injury that may result from performing these yoga poses.

Disclaimer and Terms of Use: Every effort has been made to ensure that the information in this book is accurate and complete. However, the author and publisher do not warrant the accuracy or completeness of the information, text, and graphics contained in this book. The author and publisher do not hold any responsibility for errors, omissions, or contrary interpretation of the subject matter herein. This book is presented solely for motivational, educational, and informational purposes only. This book is sold with the understanding that the author and publisher are not engaged in rendering medical, legal, or other professional advice or services. Neither the publisher or author shall be liable for damages arising herein.

Copyright 2016, by Susan Neal
Published by Christian Yoga, LLC

Unless otherwise indicated, all Scripture quotations are taken from the Holy Bible, New Living Translation, copyright © 1996, 2004, 2007, 2013 by Tyndale House Foundation. Used by permission of Tyndale House Publishers, Inc., Carol Stream, Illinois 60188. All rights reserved.

THE HOLY BIBLE, NEW INTERNATIONAL VERSION®, NIV® Copyright © 1973, 1978, 1984, 2011 by Biblica, Inc.® Used by permission. All rights reserved worldwide.

Copyright © 1995 by God's Word to the Nations. Used by permission of Baker Publishing Group

The Holy Bible, New Century Version®. Copyright © 2005 by Thomas Nelson, Inc.

Revised Standard Version of the Bible, copyright © 1946, 1952, and 1971 the Division of Christian Education of the National Council of the Churches of Christ in the United States of America. Used by permission. All rights reserved.

The Holy Bible, English Standard Version Copyright © 2001 by Crossway Bibles, a publishing ministry of Good News Publishers.

The Message (MSG) Copyright © 1993, 1994, 1995, 1996, 2000, 2001, 2002 by Eugene H. Peterson

International Standard Version (ISV) Copyright © 1995-2014 by ISV Foundation. ALL RIGHTS RESERVED INTERNATIONALLY. Used by permission of Davidson Press, LLC.

New Revised Standard Version Bible, copyright © 1989 the Division of Christian Education of the National Council of the Churches of Christ in the United States of America. Used by permission. All rights reserved.

Scripture taken from the New King James Version®. Copyright © 1982 by Thomas Nelson. Used by permission. All rights reserved.

New American Standard Bible (NASB) Copyright © 1960, 1962, 1963, 1968, 1971, 1972, 1973, 1975, 1977, 1995 by The Lockman Foundation

The Living Bible copyright © 1971 by Tyndale House Foundation. Used by permission of Tyndale House Publishers Inc., Carol Stream, Illinois 60188. All rights reserved.

ISBN-13: 978-0997763607
ISBN-10: 0997763604

Photography: RK Photos http://rkphotos1.zenfolio.com/

Cover Design: Angie Alaya

Yoga Posture Models: Susan Neal, Brooke Neal, Shelby Neal, and Callie Neal

Printed in the United States of America

Learn more information at ChristianYoga.com

Dedication: To God

Thank you for teaching me how to incorporate Scripture into yoga classes to create a Christian atmosphere. May your words in each Bible lesson be like Isaiah 55:10-11: "The rain and snow come down from the heavens and stay on the ground to water the earth. They cause the grain to grow, producing seed for the farmer and bread for the hungry. It is the same with my word. I send it out and it always produces fruit. It will accomplish all I want it to, and it will prosper everywhere I sent it."

God, thank you for showing up in the yoga pose photographs via the gleaming white cross in the background. This was unplanned by me, but planned by You!

Please access the free Scripture Yoga class, "The Fall of Lucifer" at http://christianyoga.com/free. This is a brand new theme which is not included in this book. This Bible lesson answers the questions, "Why did Lucifer fall?" and "Why do bad things happen in this world?"

An excellent aid to teaching Christian yoga classes is Scripture Yoga Cards which combine yoga poses with Bible verses. You can find the decks "How to Receive God's Peace" and "The Fruit of the Spirit" at: http://christianyoga.com/yoga-books-decks.

# Table of Contents

Introduction.................................................................................7

Chapter 1: The Journey ..............................................................9

Chapter 2: How to Memorize Scripture.....................................12

Chapter 3: How to Use Scripture Themes in Yoga Classes .........15

Chapter 4: Scripture Yoga Class Model and Poses.....................18

Chapter 5: God's Gracious Word ............................................111

Chapter 6: The Fruit of the Spirit............................................115

Chapter 7: The Greatest Gift of them all–Love ........................119

Chapter 8: How to be Filled with the Holy Spirit.....................122

Chapter 9: Don't Quench the Spirit .........................................125

Chapter 10: Temptation and the Evil One.................................128

Chapter 11: Our Advocate: The Holy Spirit .............................132

Chapter 12: How to Receive God's Peace ................................136

Chapter 13: The Great 'I AM'...................................................140

Chapter 14: The Tabernacle .....................................................144

Chapter 15: Worship and Glory ...............................................150

Chapter 16: Atonement and Righteousness ...............................152

Chapter 17: Praying and Believing...........................................156

Chapter 18: How to be God's Light and Bear His Fruit ............162

Chapter 19: Decisions, Obedience, and Joy..............................165

Chapter 20: Serving and Tithing...............................................168

Chapter 21: Marriage and Children ..........................................171

Chapter 22: God's Mighty Angels ............................................175

Chapter 23: Angelic Visitations Surrounding the Birth of Christ.................180

Chapter 24: Revelation of the Messiah through the Power of the
                    Holy Spirit.........................................................186

Chapter 25: The Lord's Festivals..............................................193

Chapter 26: Scrutiny of Yoga...................................................198

**Chapter 27: Christian Yoga Training Programs and Books** ........................203

*Notes* ................................................................................ 207
*Yoga Posture Index* ........................................................... 208
*About the Author* .............................................................. 210

# Introduction

If you are a Christian Yoga Instructor this book will save you time, impart biblical wisdom to your yoga students, and spread God's Word. For the first time, Bible lesson plans are available for Christian yoga classes. This will create the environment that a Christian is looking for in a yoga session.

Have you ever rushed off to teach a Christian yoga class and realized you had not prepared for the spiritual content of the class? You did not have the time to develop this week's theme. This book will prevent that from happening because with 21 Bible lessons specifically designed for Christian yoga classes, you will never find yourself unprepared again.

Recently, a yoga instructor attended one of my Christian yoga classes. She had been teaching Christian yoga for one year. She expressed how difficult and time-consuming it had been for her to develop a Christian theme for each of her weekly classes. I then realized many other yoga teachers could benefit from the Scripture lessons God has led me to develop, and that is why I wrote this book.

With such busy lives, we don't have time to devote four hours to each week's spiritual topic. Therefore, I have made lessons to get you out the door and prepared. Now your students will enjoy the richness of God's word without sacrificing your time. Also, your students will enjoy diverse lessons on many biblical subjects that can be applied to their lives.

The benefits of the 21 Bible lessons include:

*Saves you time

*Imparts biblical knowledge and wisdom

*Spreads God's Word

*Invokes the Holy Spirit's power

*Allows the experience of God's peace

*Draws one closer to God

I have over 30 years of experience practicing and teaching yoga. I began teaching Christian yoga in 2004. Two years later, I produced the Christian yoga DVD, *God's Mighty Angels*. At that time, there were only a handful of people who had created a Christian yoga DVD. In 2008, I created a second Christian yoga DVD, *What the Bible says about Prayer*. For more information, about these DVDs or the Scripture Yoga ministry go to ChristianYoga.com.

My prayer is this book will spread the word of God, like seeds, into many hearts, those seeds will grow 100 times beyond what is sown, and the sower (that is you) will be blessed. Matthew 13:23: "The seed that fell on good soil represents those who truly hear and understand God's word and produce a harvest of thirty, sixty, or even a hundred times as much as had been planted!"

# *Chapter 1*

# THE JOURNEY

In the 1980s, I learned to perform yoga through using the book *Richard Hittleman's Yoga: 28 Days Exercise Plan*. This book taught me each yoga posture through pictures and a thorough explanation. At the time, as a student in a dual master's program for an MBA and Master of Health Science, I needed something to decrease my stress. Yoga was extremely helpful as a stress reliever and an excellent form of exercise. I was unaware of yoga's connection with any religion since Hittleman's book made no such reference. Doing the yoga postures at home reduced the pressure I felt while working toward the completion of my Master's program.

In the 1990s, while working as an executive at Mayo Clinic Jacksonville, I started attending a yoga class twice a week to relieve work-related stress. After a year, I began to substitute for the yoga teacher, still not realizing the connection between yoga and a non-Christian belief system.

A few years later, now living in Pensacola Florida, part of the 'Bible belt,' I was teaching a weekly yoga class at a local health club when a church friend told me about 'yoga's' association with a non-Christian belief system. Really? I never encountered any references to religion in any of my yoga classes! To me, yoga was simply another form of exercise, like aerobics. Her comments were disturbing, and I became aware of the 'bad reputation' yoga had among Christians. Sadly, I have been poorly thought of by some Christians for being involved in yoga (see Chapter 26 'Scrutiny of Yoga').

Along this journey of learning, practicing, and teaching yoga, it never occurred to me that I needed to be born again and truly follow Jesus Christ. The Merriam-Webster Dictionary defines born again as "being a usually Christian person who has made a renewed or confirmed commitment of faith especially after an intense religious experience." I was raised Catholic and did not understand what being 'born again' meant until I attended my first women's retreat in 2000. During one of the worship sessions I felt Christ wrap his arms around me and through my tears I asked him to play beautiful music through me. I wanted to be his instrument in this life. So from that point on, I lived my life for God, not only for myself. Therefore, I talk to him every day and try to make his priorities my priorities. My life has been much more satisfying since that time.

After I became born again, God showed me that I love to teach, and he allowed me to do so in all sorts of ways, including Bible studies at my church. For about five years, I heard God's still small voice saying, "You need to make yoga Christian." But how? The first time the idea of teaching a 'Christian yoga' class occurred to me was in 1998. However, it was unclear how to make the yoga class appropriate for the Christian believer. Consequently, I devoted much thought and prayer toward finding a way to combine yoga and Christianity.

In 2003, while reading *The Purpose Driven Life* by Rick Warren, I accepted Rick's challenge to learn one Scripture verse per week. After learning twenty-five verses, a light bulb finally went off! How could a Christian yoga class be taught without incorporating God's Word into it? For five years, I had been waiting on God to show me how to bring Christian beliefs into the yoga class but the whole time God had been waiting for me to learn Scripture so his words could be recited during the yoga poses.

Surprisingly, but in God's perfect timing, two months later leaders at my church asked me to teach an exercise class at the church. So, in 2004, Scripture Yoga classes began! The class is still active with a faithful group of attendees. Feedback from my students has been outstanding. One of my clients Pam Antoun wrote, "Scripture based yoga has been an extremely productive use of time. Physically, I am stretching and strengthening muscles, some of which I never knew I had. Mentally, it's restful as I am simply focusing on Scripture, which is full of God's will for living a full, meaningful life. After every class, I feel spiritually nourished, well centered, and better aligned with God's will. The special breathing integrated throughout the class is extremely cleansing and refreshing. I feel like my entire body is more efficiently oxygenated and relaxed. Although I have enjoyed other yoga classes, the Scripture based yoga seems all-around more effective in improving my physical, spiritual, and mental health than any other yoga class I have attended."

During the first year I taught Scripture Yoga, throughout the class I spoke Bible verses as the Holy Spirit led. By the end of that year, I had committed more than 150 verses to memory and written them on index cards. In 2005, while attending a spiritual retreat called Emmaus Walk, the Lord directed me to gather all my Scripture cards and sort them by theme. After sorting them, there were dozens of topics. After that retreat, I taught my classes based upon a Biblical theme. There were so many themes that months could go by without teaching the same weekly lesson. It is a blessing to share these Biblical theme based lessons with you!

*Chapter 2*

# HOW TO MEMORIZE SCRIPTURE

There are many benefits of memorizing Scripture or as, Psalms 119:11 says: "hiding God's Word in our hearts." Some advantages include reducing stress, resisting temptation, hearing God speak to you, and receiving comforting reassurance of God's steadfast love. Incorporating Scripture into the yoga classes has added depth and meaning. A student once told me she quoted Bible verses she learned from Scripture Yoga during a medical procedure and it helped calm her down. Another student said she felt extremely relaxed and yet energized but at the same time connected to God and full of the Holy Spirit.

There are several steps to memorizing Scripture. First, a person needs to be inspired or motivated. Without God-given inspiration, it is difficult. So pray and ask God for the desire. For years, I thought I could not learn Bible verses because they were too challenging to remember. However, the challenge from *The Purpose Driven Life*, coupled with God's persistence and patience, motivated me even though the task seemed impossible. With prayer and God's help, the Holy Spirit empowered me to memorize many Scriptures. Philippians 4:13: "For I can do everything through Christ, who gives me strength."

A powerful way to pray is to use Scripture in prayer, essentially praying God's Word back to him. For example, "Lord, please help me learn these verses so I can recite them during yoga classes. You know my desire to obey you, learn more about you, and become closer to you. So please help me with this task, for I can do all things through Christ who gives me strength, Amen."

Next, which Scriptures should you memorize? Many times while doing a Bible study or reading the Bible, the Holy Spirit led me to learn a verse. He showed me how the verse was important personally. For example, at the stage when I was raising young children, verses on ways to discipline children were relevant and important for me to memorize.

The second step is to write the Bible verse on an index card in the following manner. Write the verse name and number at the top and bottom of the card. Then, break the verse up into short segments that are easy to memorize (Water, 1999). For example:

> John 15:16
> You didn't choose me!
> I chose you!
> I appointed you
> to go and
> produce lovely fruit always.
> John 15:16

This simple and effective method makes it easy to learn one line of the verse at a time. Continue to do this until the entire verse is memorized. For me, it was harder to learn the verse name and number than the verse itself. That is why I wrote the verse name and number at the beginning and the end of the verse.

To remember a Bible verse, it is important to review it on a weekly basis. I would study the Scripture cards when I worked out at the gym. My husband thought this was a very creative way to exercise my body, mind, and spirit through the word of God. This weekly repetition kept the verse at the forefront of my mind. You could bring the Scripture cards with you when you walk or tape one to your bathroom mirror, or keep them in your purse and review them when you can. Be creative!

Chapters 5-25 include the 21 theme-based Bible lessons for a Scripture Yoga class. In addition to this book, I created Scripture Yoga Cards that have yoga poses and Scripture verses on them. You can purchase them on ChristianYoga.com. These cards would simplify the preparation for each of your classes.

Sign up to be notified when a new deck of Scripture Yoga Cards become available and receive the free Scripture Yoga class, "The Fall of Lucifer" at with http://christianyoga.com/free. This is a brand new theme which is not included in this book. This Bible lesson answers the questions, "Why did Lucifer fall?" and "Why do bad things happen in this world?"

Otherwise, you could make copies of the Scriptures and put them on index cards. Either place a rubber band on the cards or hole punch each one and put a key ring on the group to keep them together. Both methods work well. For each yoga theme, number the index cards in case they get out of order. Bring these Scripture cards with you to your exercise class.

Each Scripture Yoga class is like teaching a mini Bible study. So, the verses are arranged purposefully and progressively depending on the topic. I can go for months without reusing the same theme and now you can too!

*Chapter 3*

# HOW TO USE SCRIPTURE THEMES IN YOGA CLASSES

Store the 21 Bible lesson index cards, in a specific order, in a drawer so you know which ones have recently been used. Before a yoga class, take out the top two sets of cards and pray, asking God to direct you about which topic to use, and to help you during the class. For the chosen subject, review all the Scriptures before the class.

It is important to invoke the power of the Holy Spirit before and during your class. Therefore, at the beginning of each yoga session, pray with the participants and inform them of the title of the biblical theme for that day. The index cards can lie beside your yoga mat so you can refer to them throughout the class. Many times, the Holy Spirit has inspired me to add a story relevant to the topic.

For example, I may have heard something on the radio or at a Bible study or recall a situation within my family. These everyday life examples enhance the depth of the class, and the participants enjoy the authenticity and openness. As teachers, it is important to share our faults. We are not perfect people, and when appropriate we can share when we've messed up and how the Lord has come to our aid. Be genuine and lay before the participants your heart and desire to please God. This makes the instructor a real person who is approachable and hopefully humble.

Be open to the urges you may receive from the Holy Spirit during the yoga sessions. Many times the Holy Spirit will lead me to repeat one individual Scripture verse several times throughout the class. This creates a central idea for the yoga participant. For example, when using the yoga theme titled God's Gracious Word, I usually repeat the following verse several times: Acts 20:32 (The Message) "God whose gracious Word can make you into what he wants you to be and give you everything you could possibly need." At the beginning of the relaxation portion of the class, I repeat this same verse to give the participants the word of God to ponder during their few minutes of relaxation.

In some classes you will feel the leading of the Holy Spirit and other times you will not. Maybe you won't feel the Spirit's leading when you are sick, or too much is going on in your life, or you have unconfessed sin. Realize this is normal. Pray and ask for God's help and guidance before, during, and after your class. Many times in my opening prayer I will ask God to lead me to the things he wants me to say.

What type of music should you use? Many Christian yoga instructors use Christian music. However, to me, there is much more to making the yoga class Christian than just adding Christian music. I use classical piano music. My favorite CD is *After the Rain* by Michael Jones. I have always enjoyed listening to a soothing piano melody. I tried all sorts of different types of music, but background piano music has worked best for my classes since I speak Scripture verses throughout the class. However, during some yoga postures I am quiet and allow the participant to spend time with God, especially after I have recited a thought provoking verse.

The 21 Bible lessons included in chapters 5-25 provide a structured format for you to use during your yoga sessions, but you can add or delete Scriptures to the topic as the Holy Spirit leads you. Choose themes that speak to you and select those to recite during your classes. Of course, you could create your own Scripture class based upon what God places on your heart.

Sign up to be notified when a new deck of Scripture Yoga Cards become available at http://christianyoga.com/free and receive a free gift.

Many versions and translations of the Bible are available. However, the primary one I have used for the Scripture Yoga class has been the *New Living Translation*. The most important thing is getting the meaning of the verse across in the most understandable language. Therefore, I would suggest looking at several versions of the Bible before deciding which one to use. BlueLetterBible.org or Logos Software is very helpful. Many times only part of a verse may be used which would be indicated by 'a' or 'b' by the Bible verse. The 'a' represents the first half of the verse, and the 'b' is the second half. This keeps the Bible verse short while getting across the theme of the yoga class. For your information, *The Living Bible* (LB) and *The Message* are paraphrased and not direct translations.

Recite the Scripture verses while holding the yoga postures. Try to hold most poses for 3-4 breaths; this should be an adequate amount of time to recite a Bible verse. You can choose to repeat a verse again or say it only once. You can quote a Scripture during every posture or only a few; it is totally up to you and how the Holy Spirit leads you. I usually leave the last Bible verse for the relaxation time or repeat it again at that time. The next chapter is an example of my class format, and it gives specific instructions about how and when to recite the Scriptures. The Scripture Yoga Cards have the verse corresponding with a specific yoga pose, so it is already assembled for you.

Let's pray: God, please bless my endeavor of pouring your Word into my participants' hearts. May it be as said in Proverbs 2:6: "For the Lord grants wisdom! His every word is a treasure of knowledge and understanding." Lord may this be so as your Word is proclaimed, Amen.

# Chapter 4

# SCRIPTURE YOGA CLASS MODEL AND POSES

I teach a gentle, beginner-intermediate yoga class. Listed below are three different yoga class sessions for 60-75 minute classes. I begin my classes with 15-20 minutes of stretching poses to loosen up all the muscles in the body. Be sure to perform a series of warm-up stretches, as indicated in this class outline, before beginning the more difficult yoga postures. This will decrease the possibility of injury. Be watchful of your students and modify poses as needed. As with any fitness routine be sure to have participants check with a doctor before performing these yoga postures.

In addition, a posture index is included at the back of this book to use as a reference.

**Gentle Yoga Posture Session**

Cross Legged
Chin to Chest
Ear to Shoulder
Head Turns
Son (Sun) Breath
Upper Body Stretching
Elbow to Knee
Seated Open-Angle Pose/Forward Bend
Seated Open-Angle Side Bend

Revolved Head-to-Knee Pose
Butterfly
Bent Knee Seated Forward Fold
Seated Forward Bend
Seated Spinal Twist
Lion
Table
Cat and Dog Stretch
Thread the Needle
Pigeon

Yoga Mudra

Cleansing Breath

Squat

Standing Forward Bend

Mountain

Half Moon Side Bend

Standing Abdominal Lifts

Warrior I

Triangle

Tree

Half-Locust

Cobra

Locust

Bow

Child's Pose

Double Leg Raises

Supine Reach Through (Variation)

Bridge

Shoulder Stand

Fish

Lying Spinal Twist (One Leg Variation)

Alternate Nostril Breath

Corpse Pose

Knee Hug

**Intermediate I Yoga Posture Session** (same as gentle series except)

Add Shoulder Shrug/Circles

Add Staff Pose

Add Camel

Add Kegel

Standing Side Yoga Mudra instead of kneeling Yoga Mudra

Warrior II instead of Triangle

Warrior III instead of Tree

Boat instead of Double Leg Raises

Single Knee Hug instead of Knee Hug

**Intermediate II Yoga Posture Session** (same as gentle series except)

Cow Face instead of Thread the Needle

Add Low Lunge

Add Downward Dog

Add Plank

Add Standing Forward Bend with Leg Clasp and Halfway Lift

Posture Clasp instead of sitting Yoga Mudra

Eagle or Dancer instead of Tree

Sun Salutation instead of Warrior I and Triangle

Add Wheel (if applicable for your class level)

Reclining Spinal Twist (Two Knee Variation) instead of Lying Spinal Twist

**Yoga Posture Modification Suggestion**

Cross-legged pose-extend the legs in front of you while bending your knees instead of crossing your legs.

Downward Dog-move into the Half Dog where you stay on your knees and forearms while lifting your tailbone up.

Camel-from a kneeling position, sit on your heels and place your palms flat on the floor behind you with fingertips pointed away from your body. Lift your pelvis so you have a straight line between your knees, neck, and head.

Dancer-stand in front of a wall so your fingertips touch the wall as you lean forward into the pose.

Cobra-keep your forearms on the mat while moving your upper torso up. This modified Cobra is called the Sphinx pose.

Plank-keep your forearms on the mat when moving into the Plank. This decreases the pressure on your wrists.

Bridge-stay in the basic pose of the Bridge, therefore, you do not clasp your hands together under your back.

Shoulder Stand-only lift your legs up into the air, not your pelvis. Then perform the ankle movements.

Fish-do not tilt your head back, instead stay in the basic posture of the Fish with your upper torso weight on your elbows.

Begin your class with prayer: "Lord, thank you for this time together. Please bless the individuals represented here. Help us to draw closer to you and focus on your word. Through Jesus' name we pray, Amen."

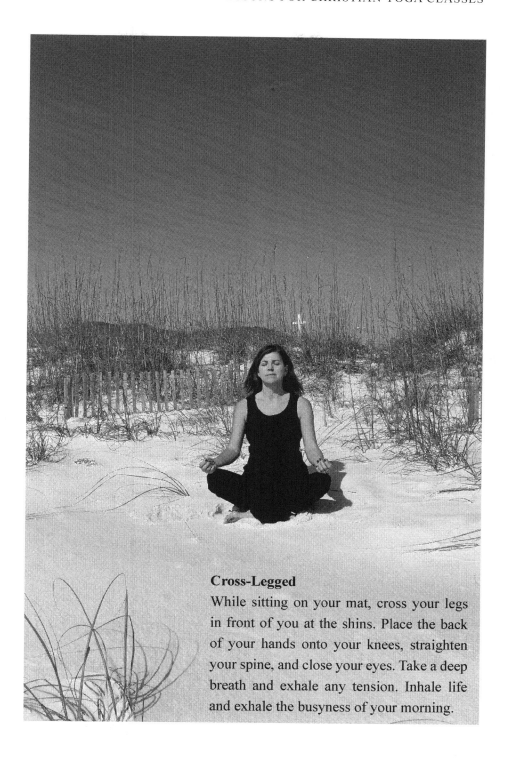

## Cross-Legged

While sitting on your mat, cross your legs in front of you at the shins. Place the back of your hands onto your knees, straighten your spine, and close your eyes. Take a deep breath and exhale any tension. Inhale life and exhale the busyness of your morning.

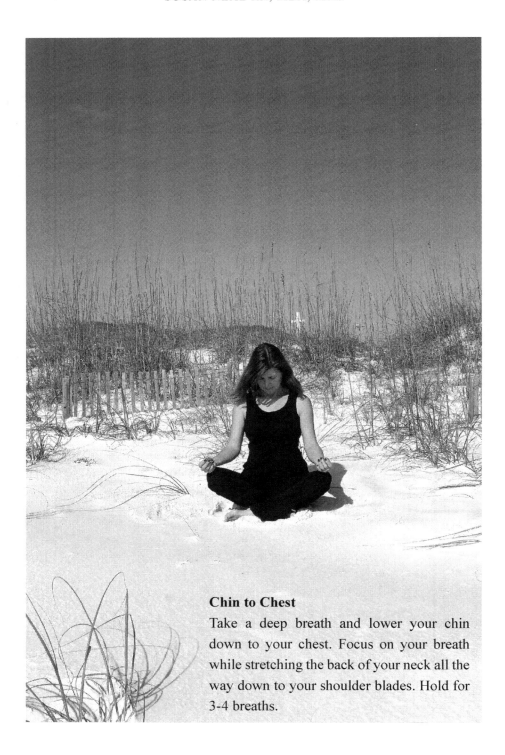

**Chin to Chest**

Take a deep breath and lower your chin down to your chest. Focus on your breath while stretching the back of your neck all the way down to your shoulder blades. Hold for 3-4 breaths.

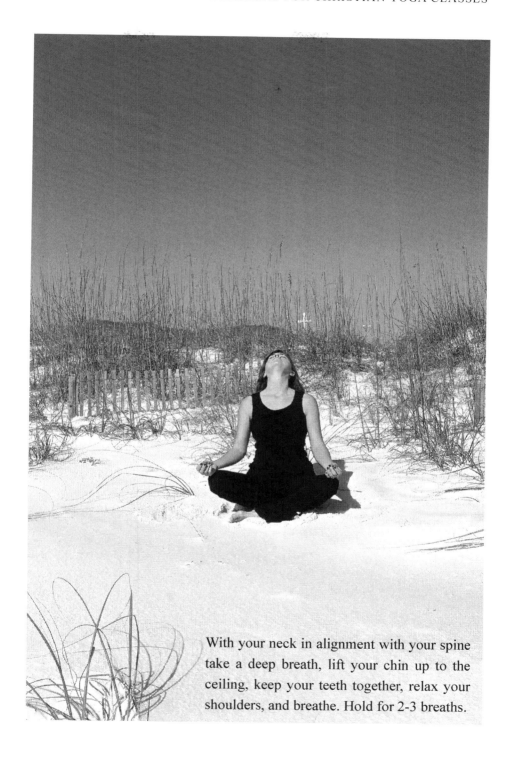

With your neck in alignment with your spine take a deep breath, lift your chin up to the ceiling, keep your teeth together, relax your shoulders, and breathe. Hold for 2-3 breaths.

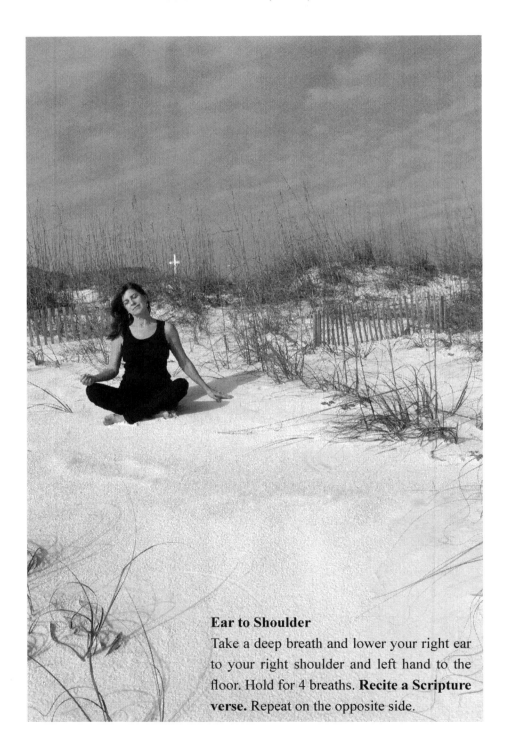

**Ear to Shoulder**

Take a deep breath and lower your right ear to your right shoulder and left hand to the floor. Hold for 4 breaths. **Recite a Scripture verse.** Repeat on the opposite side.

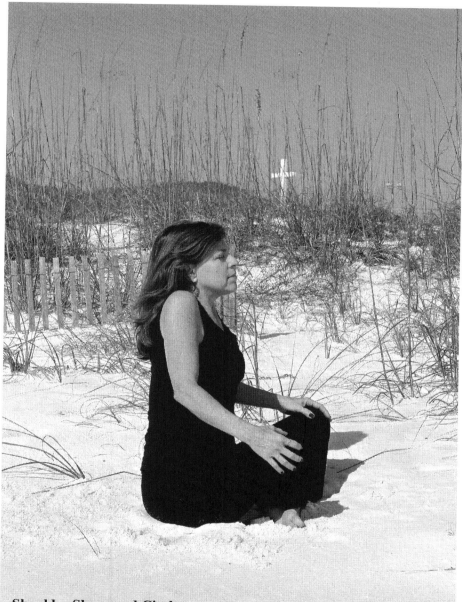

## Shoulder Shrug and Circles

Inhale and lift your shoulders up toward your ears. Exhale and lower the shoulders. Repeat several times. Inhale and raise your shoulders toward your ears and rotate them forward in large circles and backward in circles.

Feel how good it feels to stretch all the muscles in your neck. Now is a time to quiet your mind and listen to the Word of God, allowing these words to enter your heart and bloom like flowers in Springtime.

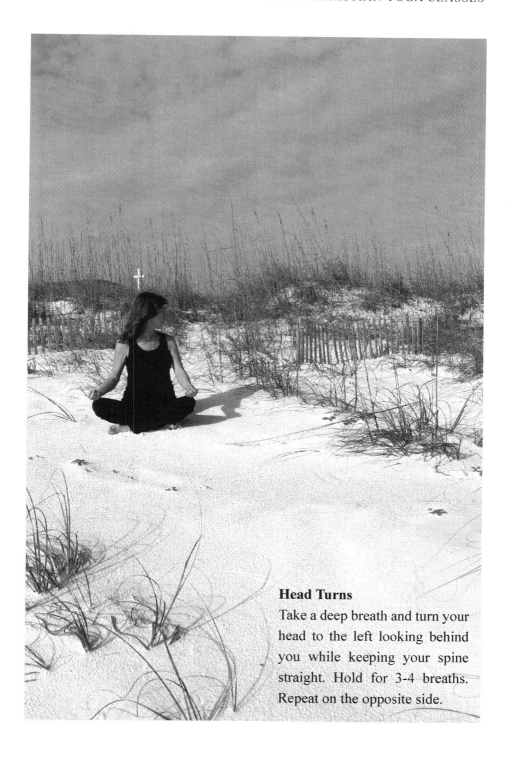

**Head Turns**

Take a deep breath and turn your head to the left looking behind you while keeping your spine straight. Hold for 3-4 breaths. Repeat on the opposite side.

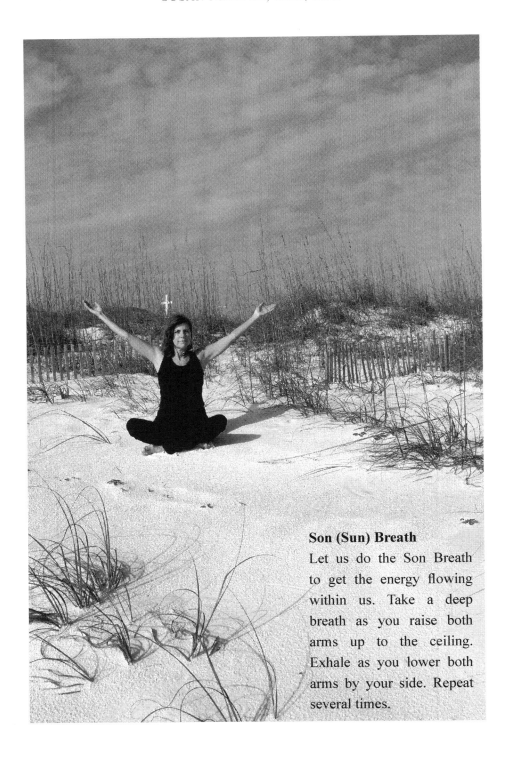

**Son (Sun) Breath**

Let us do the Son Breath to get the energy flowing within us. Take a deep breath as you raise both arms up to the ceiling. Exhale as you lower both arms by your side. Repeat several times.

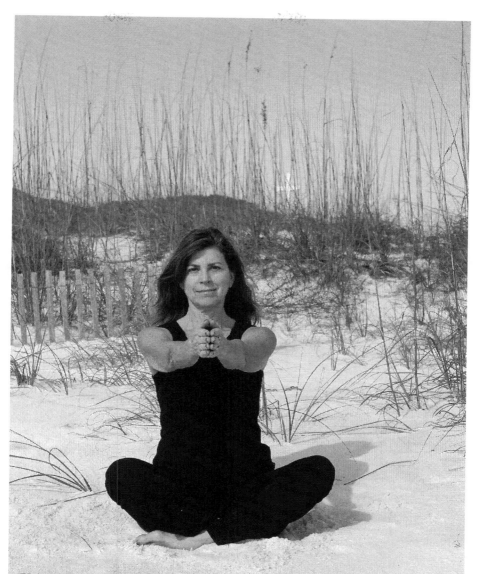

## Upper Body Stretching

Now we will stretch our upper body. On an inhale, put your hands together in prayer position in front of your chest. Exhale, move your arms out in front of you, elbows straight, hands in a prayer position. Straighten your spine and neck, stretch through your shoulders, elbows, hands, and fingertips. **Recite a Scripture verse.**

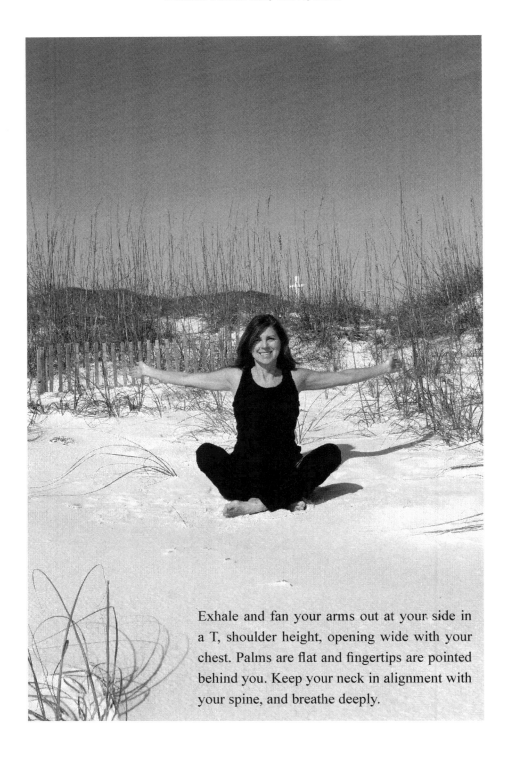

Exhale and fan your arms out at your side in a T, shoulder height, opening wide with your chest. Palms are flat and fingertips are pointed behind you. Keep your neck in alignment with your spine, and breathe deeply.

Remember to inhale and exhale deeply during all of the yoga postures. Many times we take a shallow breath. During this yoga class, focus on expanding your lungs fully like a balloon and exhaling completely.

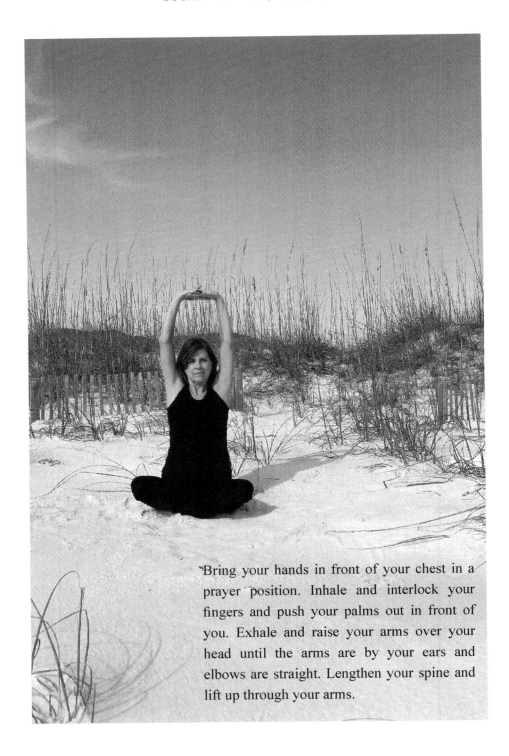

Bring your hands in front of your chest in a prayer position. Inhale and interlock your fingers and push your palms out in front of you. Exhale and raise your arms over your head until the arms are by your ears and elbows are straight. Lengthen your spine and lift up through your arms.

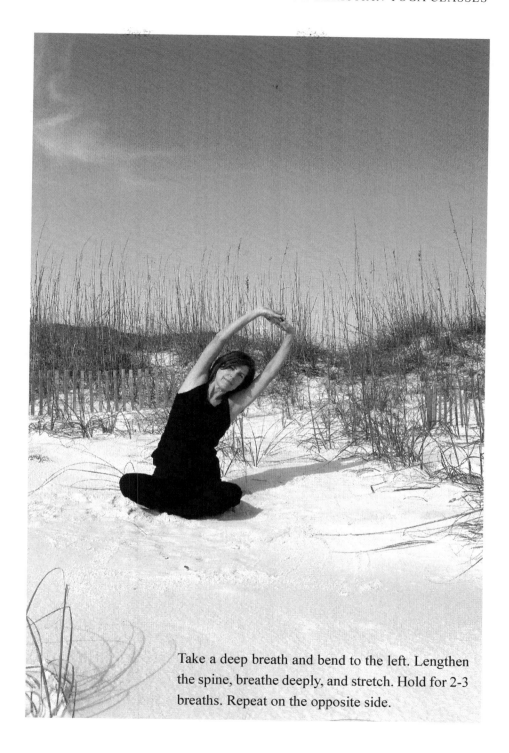

Take a deep breath and bend to the left. Lengthen the spine, breathe deeply, and stretch. Hold for 2-3 breaths. Repeat on the opposite side.

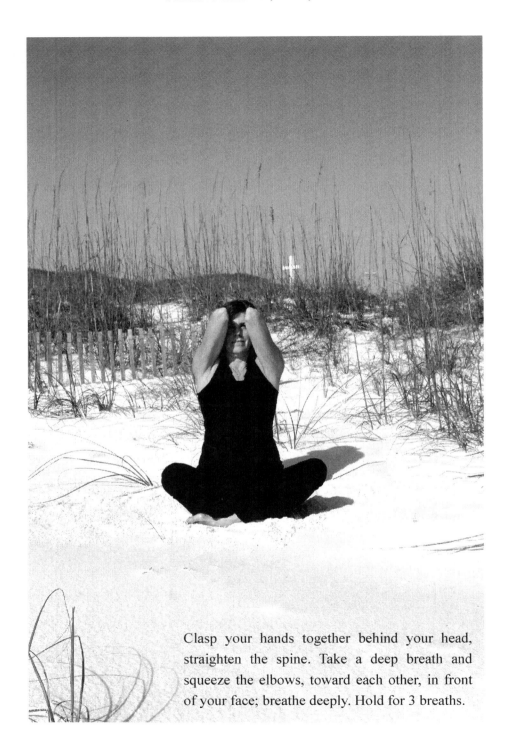

Clasp your hands together behind your head, straighten the spine. Take a deep breath and squeeze the elbows, toward each other, in front of your face; breathe deeply. Hold for 3 breaths.

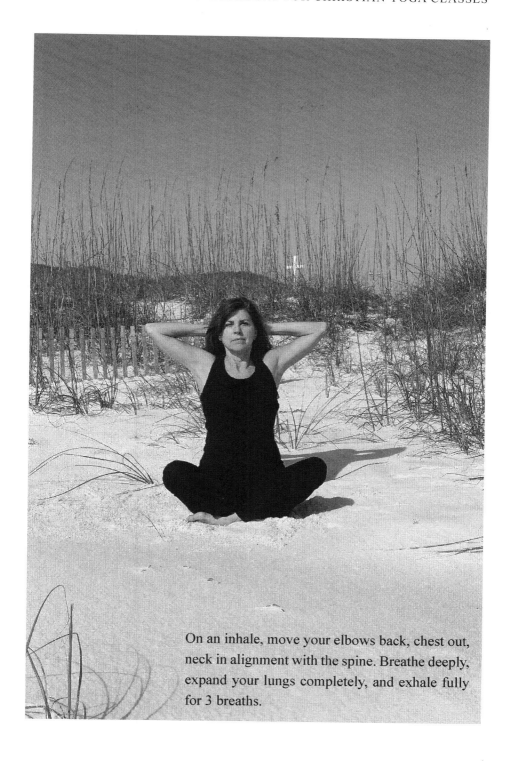

On an inhale, move your elbows back, chest out, neck in alignment with the spine. Breathe deeply, expand your lungs completely, and exhale fully for 3 breaths.

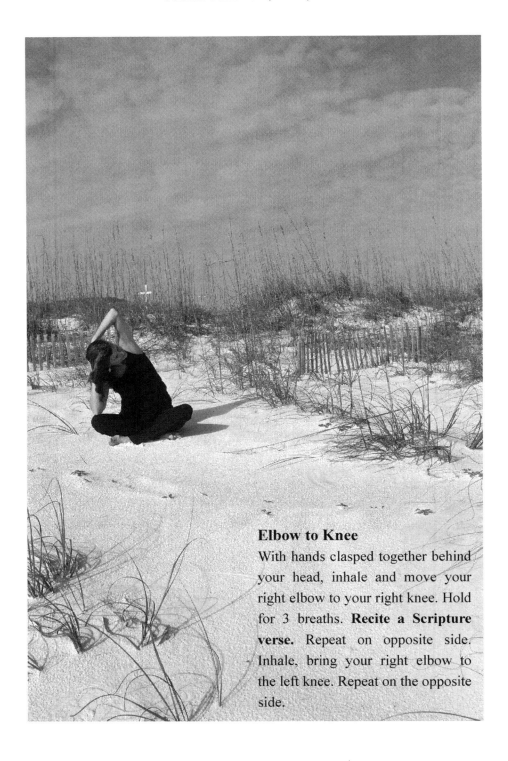

## Elbow to Knee

With hands clasped together behind your head, inhale and move your right elbow to your right knee. Hold for 3 breaths. **Recite a Scripture verse.** Repeat on opposite side. Inhale, bring your right elbow to the left knee. Repeat on the opposite side.

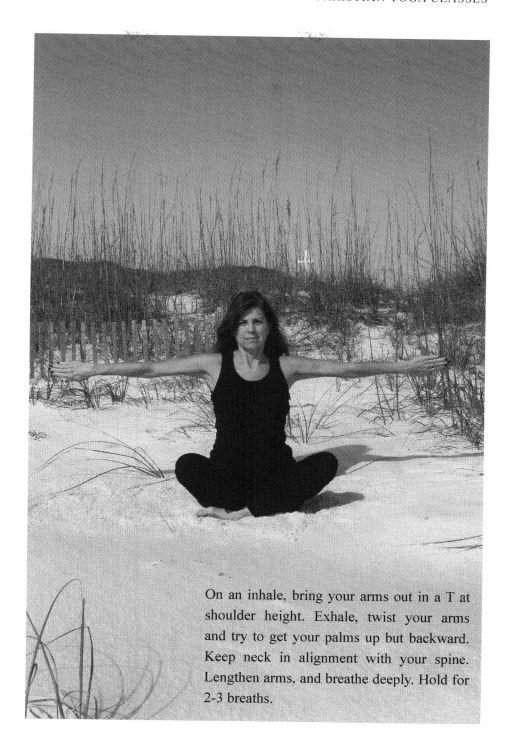

On an inhale, bring your arms out in a T at shoulder height. Exhale, twist your arms and try to get your palms up but backward. Keep neck in alignment with your spine. Lengthen arms, and breathe deeply. Hold for 2-3 breaths.

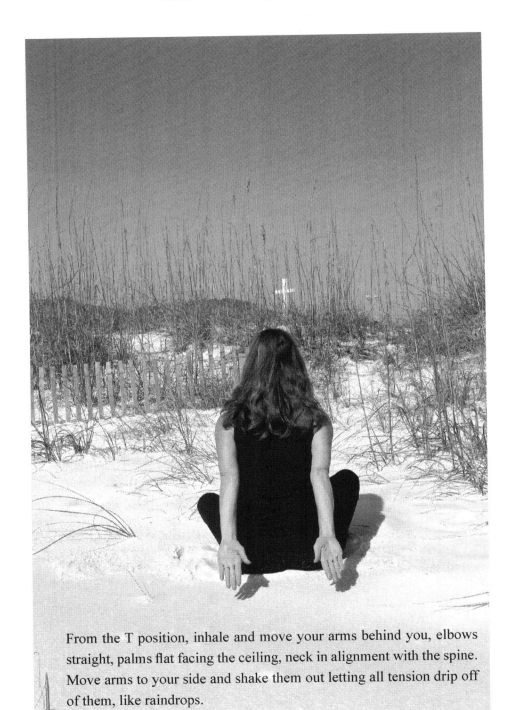

From the T position, inhale and move your arms behind you, elbows straight, palms flat facing the ceiling, neck in alignment with the spine. Move arms to your side and shake them out letting all tension drip off of them, like raindrops.

**Cross-Legged**

While sitting on your mat, cross your legs in front of you at the shins. Place your hands onto your knees, close your eyes and feel how good it feels to stretch the muscles in your neck, shoulders, arms, all the way down to your hands and fingertips. Now we will stretch our lower body as we have our upper body.

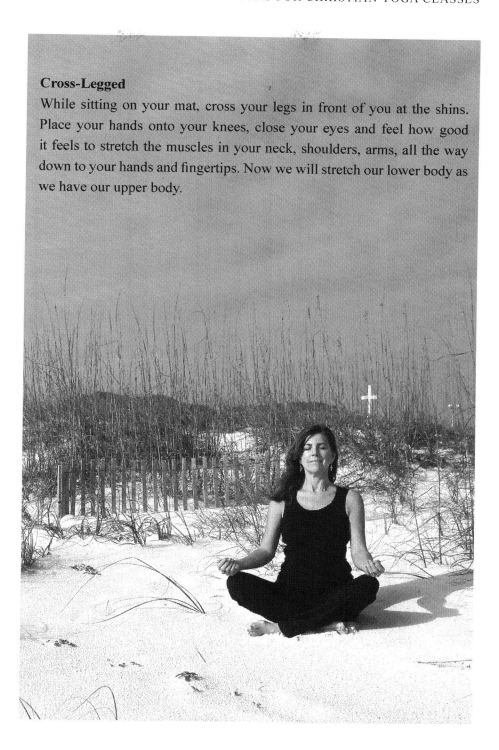

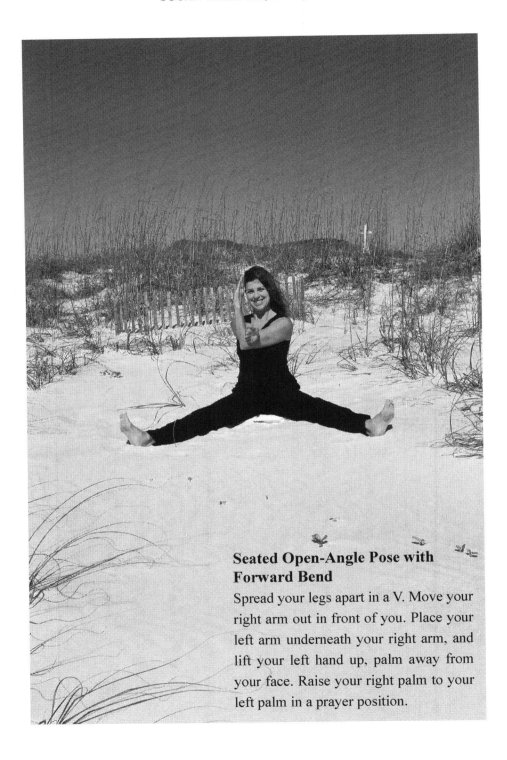

## Seated Open-Angle Pose with Forward Bend

Spread your legs apart in a V. Move your right arm out in front of you. Place your left arm underneath your right arm, and lift your left hand up, palm away from your face. Raise your right palm to your left palm in a prayer position.

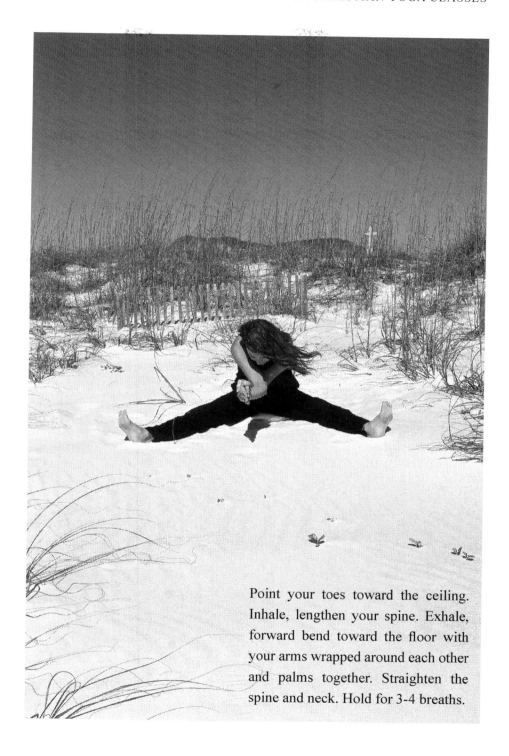

Point your toes toward the ceiling. Inhale, lengthen your spine. Exhale, forward bend toward the floor with your arms wrapped around each other and palms together. Straighten the spine and neck. Hold for 3-4 breaths.

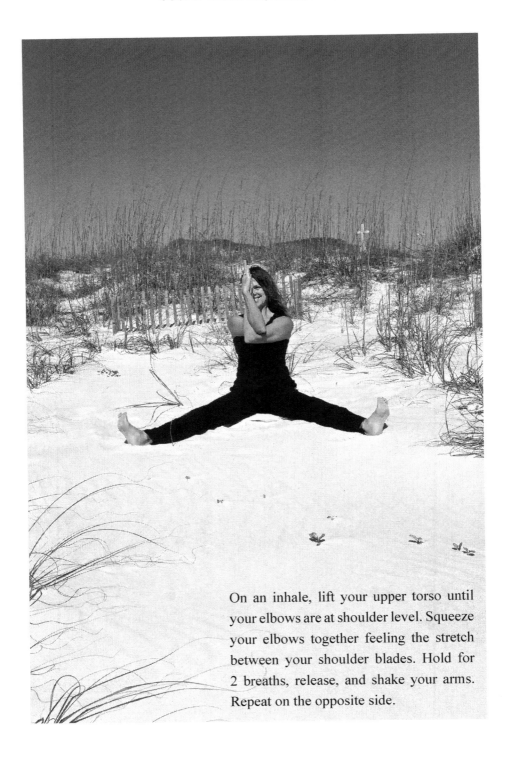

On an inhale, lift your upper torso until your elbows are at shoulder level. Squeeze your elbows together feeling the stretch between your shoulder blades. Hold for 2 breaths, release, and shake your arms. Repeat on the opposite side.

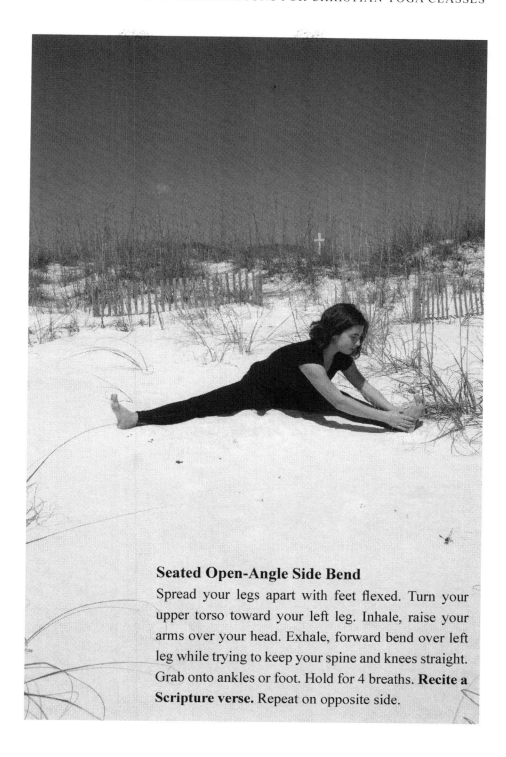

### Seated Open-Angle Side Bend

Spread your legs apart with feet flexed. Turn your upper torso toward your left leg. Inhale, raise your arms over your head. Exhale, forward bend over left leg while trying to keep your spine and knees straight. Grab onto ankles or foot. Hold for 4 breaths. **Recite a Scripture verse.** Repeat on opposite side.

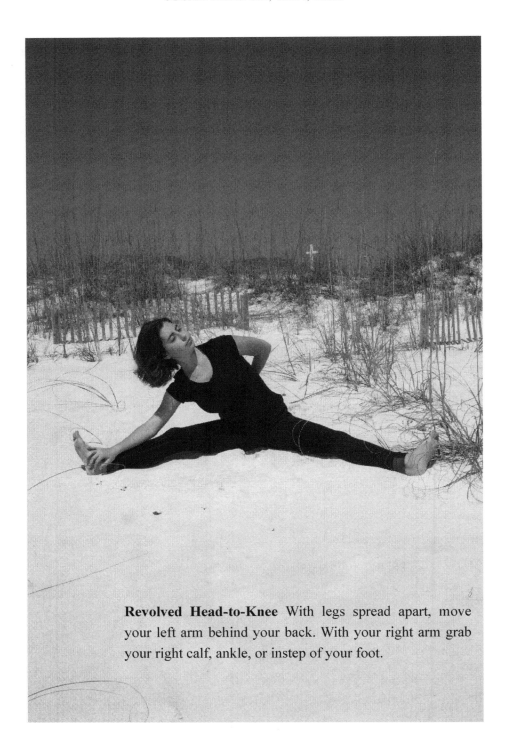

**Revolved Head-to-Knee** With legs spread apart, move your left arm behind your back. With your right arm grab your right calf, ankle, or instep of your foot.

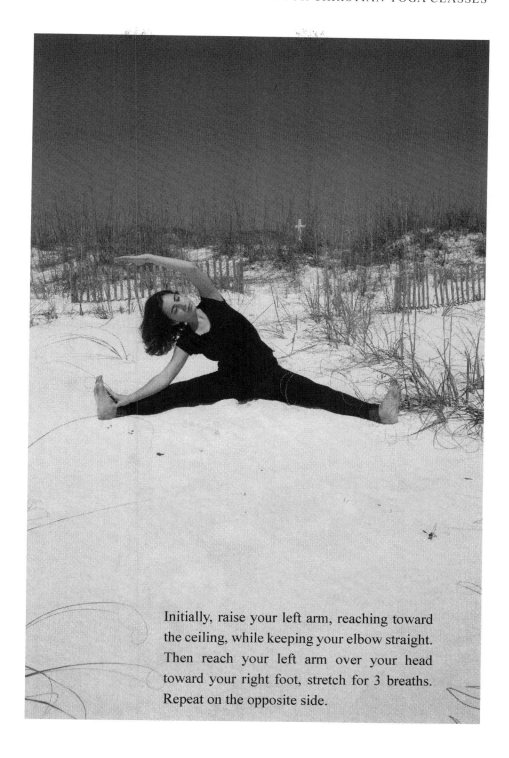

Initially, raise your left arm, reaching toward the ceiling, while keeping your elbow straight. Then reach your left arm over your head toward your right foot, stretch for 3 breaths. Repeat on the opposite side.

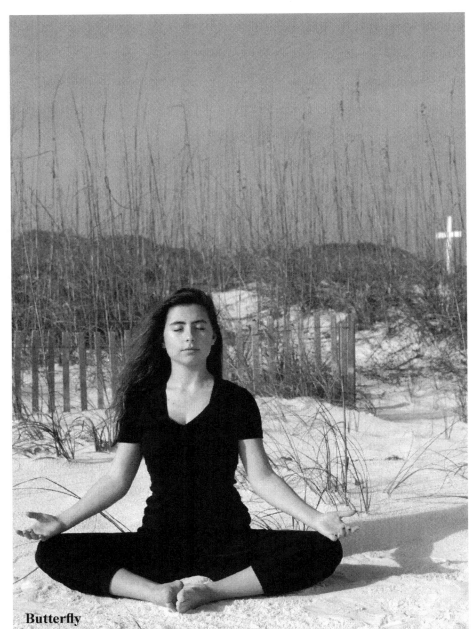

**Butterfly**
Put your feet together and flutter your knees. Inhale, lengthen your spine and neck; exhale, lower your knees down toward the floor and hold for 3 breaths.

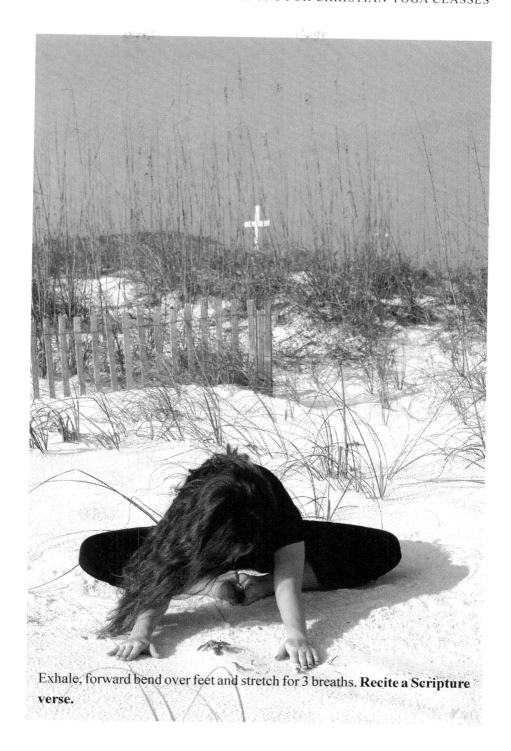

Exhale, forward bend over feet and stretch for 3 breaths. **Recite a Scripture verse.**

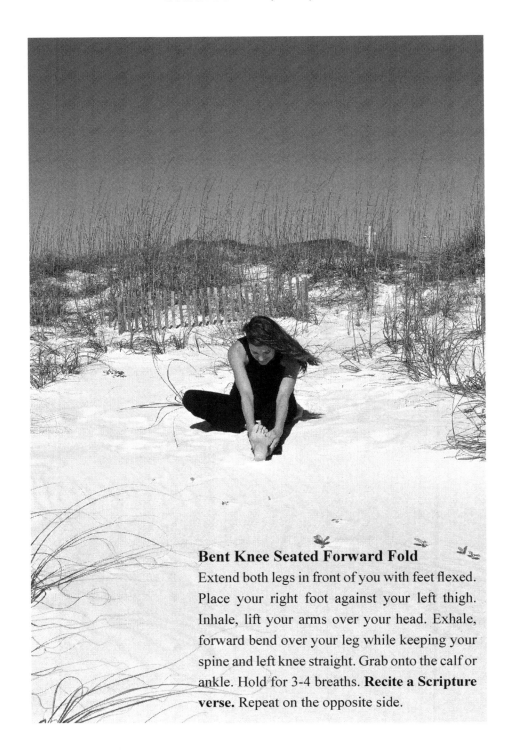

**Bent Knee Seated Forward Fold**
Extend both legs in front of you with feet flexed.
Place your right foot against your left thigh.
Inhale, lift your arms over your head. Exhale,
forward bend over your leg while keeping your
spine and left knee straight. Grab onto the calf or
ankle. Hold for 3-4 breaths. **Recite a Scripture
verse.** Repeat on the opposite side.

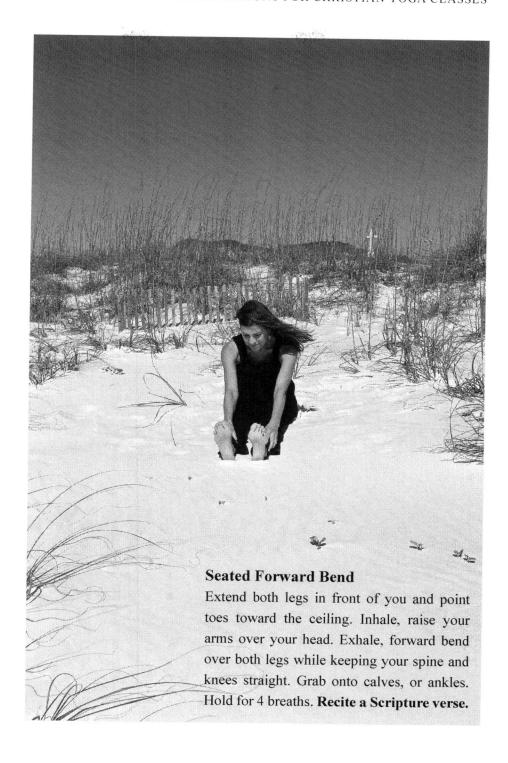

### Seated Forward Bend

Extend both legs in front of you and point toes toward the ceiling. Inhale, raise your arms over your head. Exhale, forward bend over both legs while keeping your spine and knees straight. Grab onto calves, or ankles. Hold for 4 breaths. **Recite a Scripture verse.**

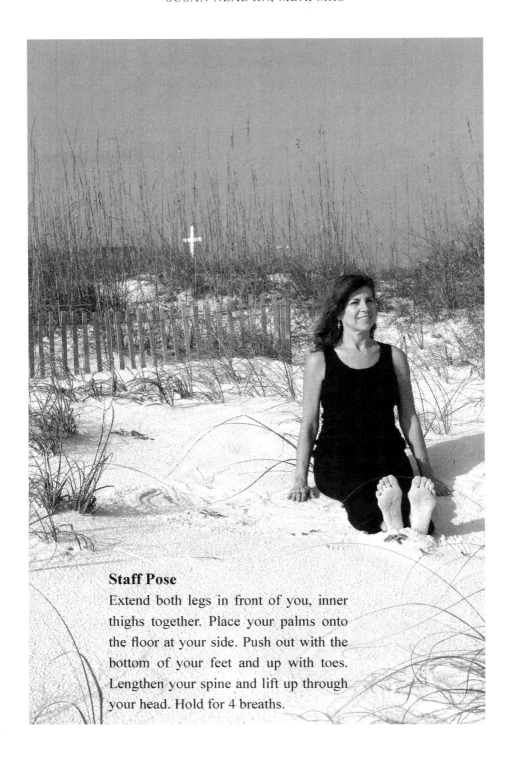

**Staff Pose**

Extend both legs in front of you, inner thighs together. Place your palms onto the floor at your side. Push out with the bottom of your feet and up with toes. Lengthen your spine and lift up through your head. Hold for 4 breaths.

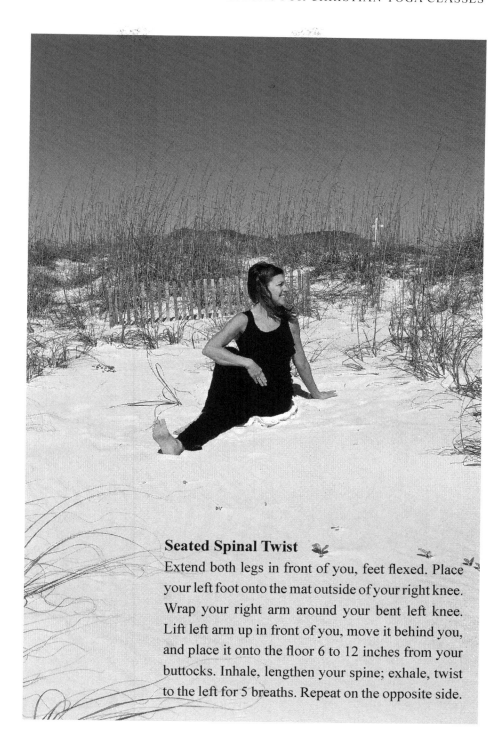

### Seated Spinal Twist

Extend both legs in front of you, feet flexed. Place your left foot onto the mat outside of your right knee. Wrap your right arm around your bent left knee. Lift left arm up in front of you, move it behind you, and place it onto the floor 6 to 12 inches from your buttocks. Inhale, lengthen your spine; exhale, twist to the left for 5 breaths. Repeat on the opposite side.

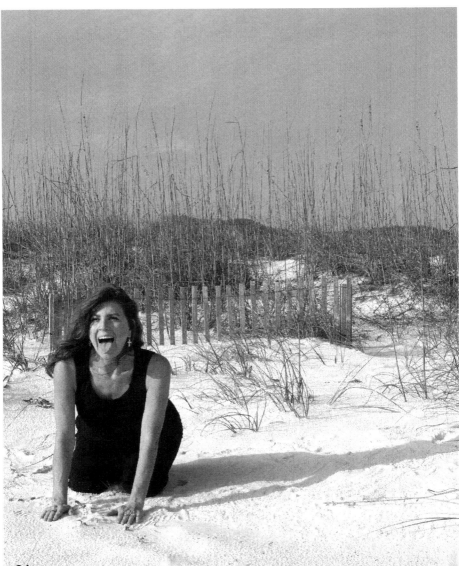

**Lion**

It is important to stretch the muscles in your face as well as the rest of your body. Sit on your heels, spread your hands and place them onto the floor in front of you. Open your mouth, extend tongue, widen eyes, and stretch all the muscles in your face. Hold for 4-6 breaths, and then roar like God's mighty Lion of Judah!

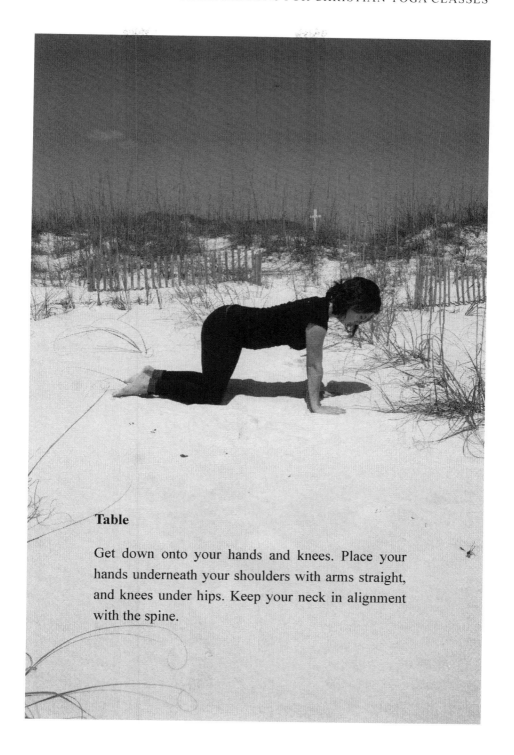

## Table

Get down onto your hands and knees. Place your hands underneath your shoulders with arms straight, and knees under hips. Keep your neck in alignment with the spine.

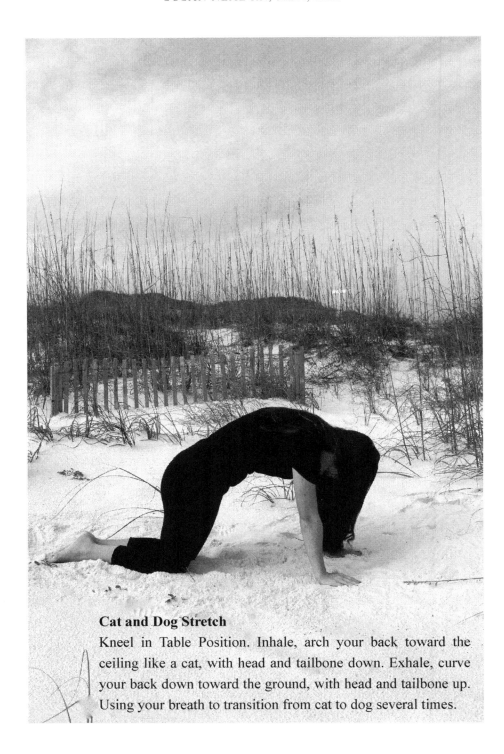

**Cat and Dog Stretch**

Kneel in Table Position. Inhale, arch your back toward the ceiling like a cat, with head and tailbone down. Exhale, curve your back down toward the ground, with head and tailbone up. Using your breath to transition from cat to dog several times.

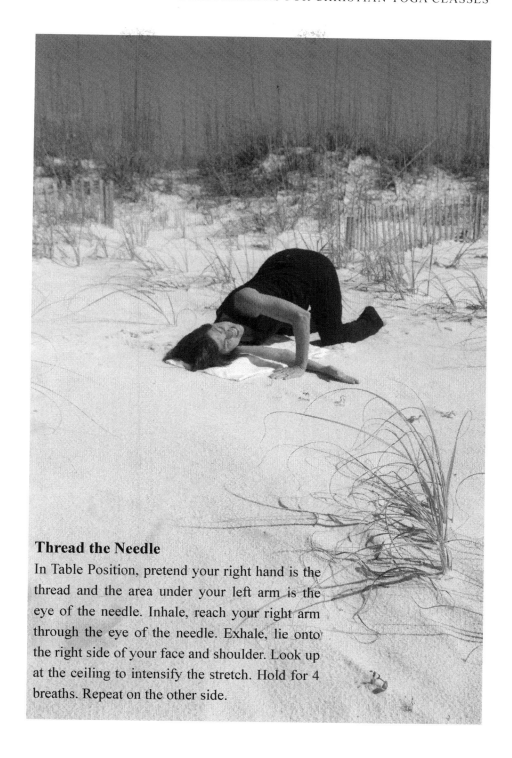

## Thread the Needle

In Table Position, pretend your right hand is the thread and the area under your left arm is the eye of the needle. Inhale, reach your right arm through the eye of the needle. Exhale, lie onto the right side of your face and shoulder. Look up at the ceiling to intensify the stretch. Hold for 4 breaths. Repeat on the other side.

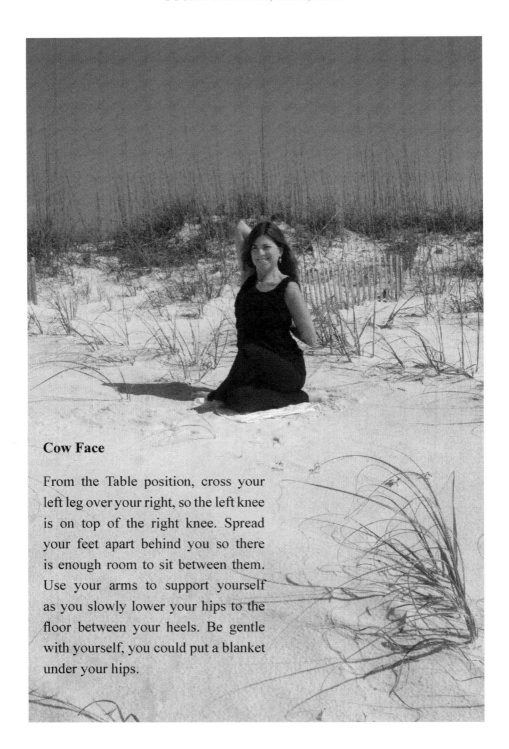

## Cow Face

From the Table position, cross your left leg over your right, so the left knee is on top of the right knee. Spread your feet apart behind you so there is enough room to sit between them. Use your arms to support yourself as you slowly lower your hips to the floor between your heels. Be gentle with yourself, you could put a blanket under your hips.

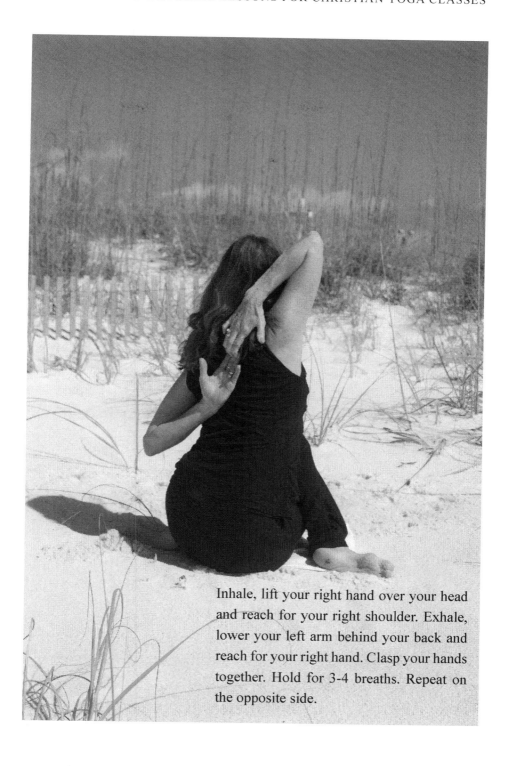

Inhale, lift your right hand over your head and reach for your right shoulder. Exhale, lower your left arm behind your back and reach for your right hand. Clasp your hands together. Hold for 3-4 breaths. Repeat on the opposite side.

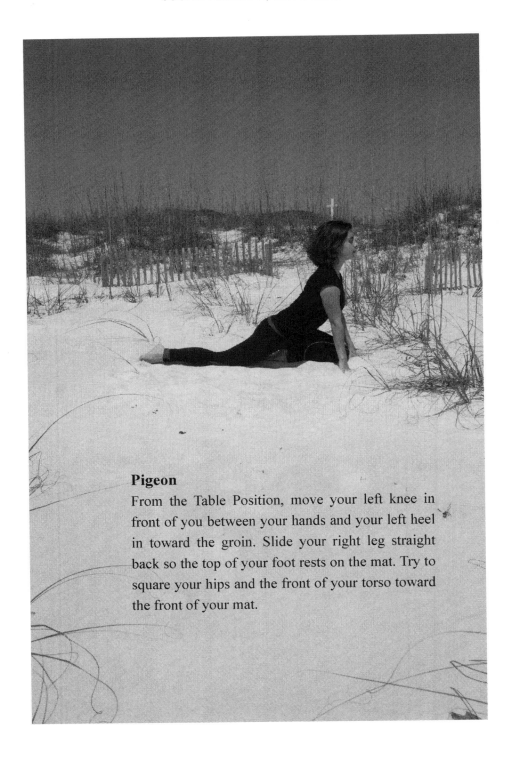

**Pigeon**

From the Table Position, move your left knee in front of you between your hands and your left heel in toward the groin. Slide your right leg straight back so the top of your foot rests on the mat. Try to square your hips and the front of your torso toward the front of your mat.

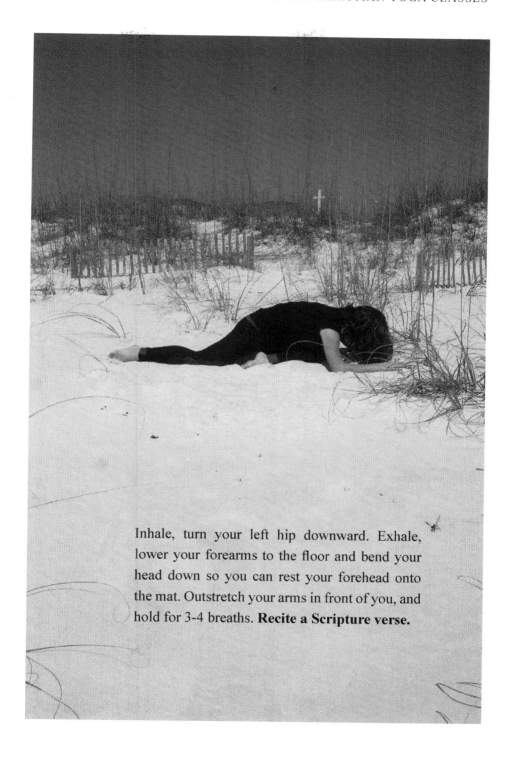

Inhale, turn your left hip downward. Exhale, lower your forearms to the floor and bend your head down so you can rest your forehead onto the mat. Outstretch your arms in front of you, and hold for 3-4 breaths. **Recite a Scripture verse.**

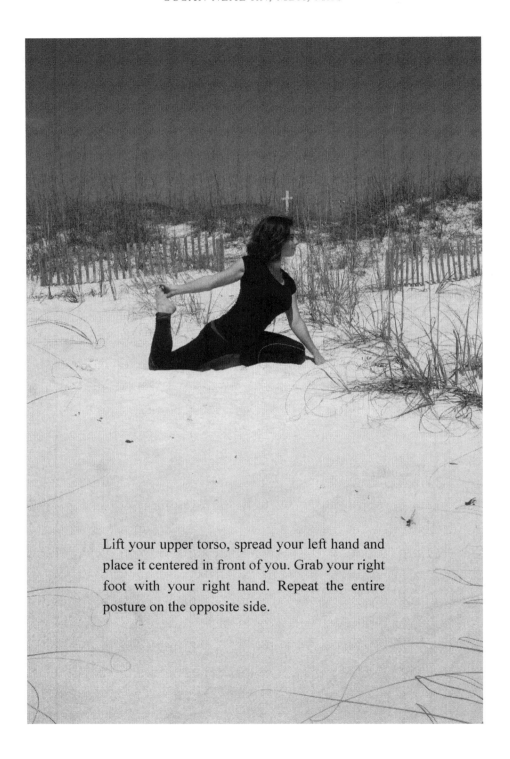

Lift your upper torso, spread your left hand and place it centered in front of you. Grab your right foot with your right hand. Repeat the entire posture on the opposite side.

## Downward Dog

From Table position, curl your toes into the floor. Exhale, lift your bottom up toward the ceiling. Straighten your elbows and back while keeping your neck in alignment with the spine. Press your chest toward your knees.

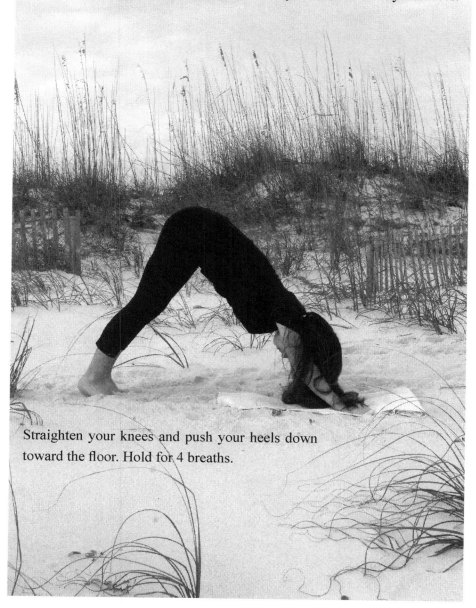

Straighten your knees and push your heels down toward the floor. Hold for 4 breaths.

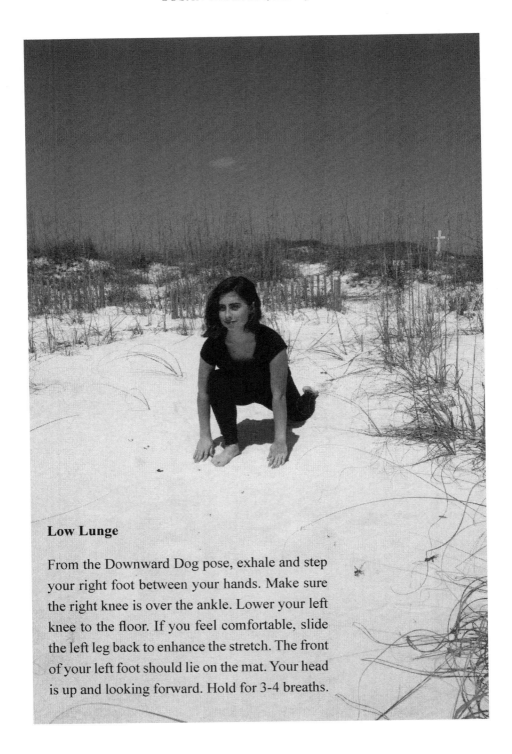

## Low Lunge

From the Downward Dog pose, exhale and step your right foot between your hands. Make sure the right knee is over the ankle. Lower your left knee to the floor. If you feel comfortable, slide the left leg back to enhance the stretch. The front of your left foot should lie on the mat. Your head is up and looking forward. Hold for 3-4 breaths.

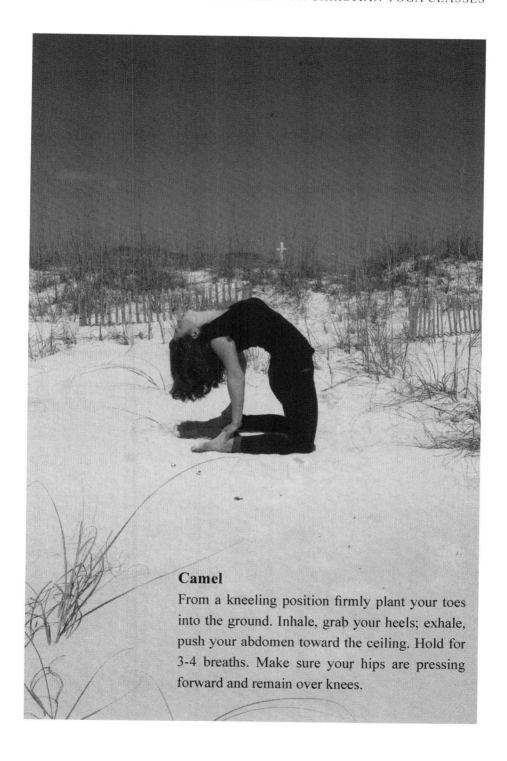

## Camel

From a kneeling position firmly plant your toes into the ground. Inhale, grab your heels; exhale, push your abdomen toward the ceiling. Hold for 3-4 breaths. Make sure your hips are pressing forward and remain over knees.

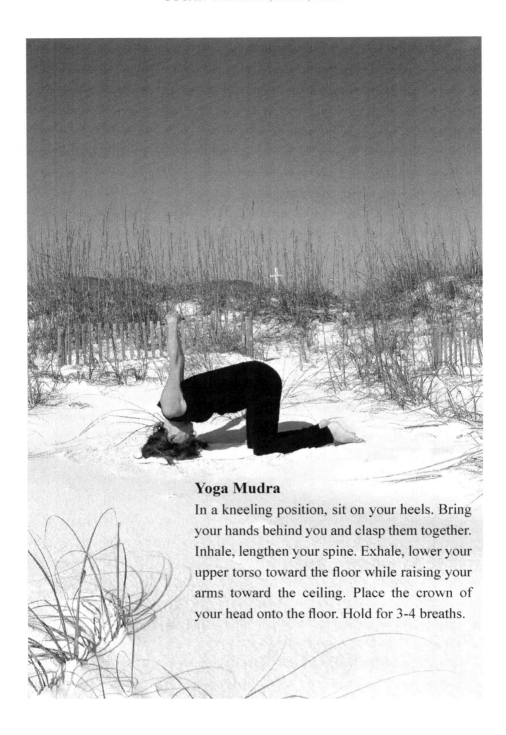

### Yoga Mudra

In a kneeling position, sit on your heels. Bring your hands behind you and clasp them together. Inhale, lengthen your spine. Exhale, lower your upper torso toward the floor while raising your arms toward the ceiling. Place the crown of your head onto the floor. Hold for 3-4 breaths.

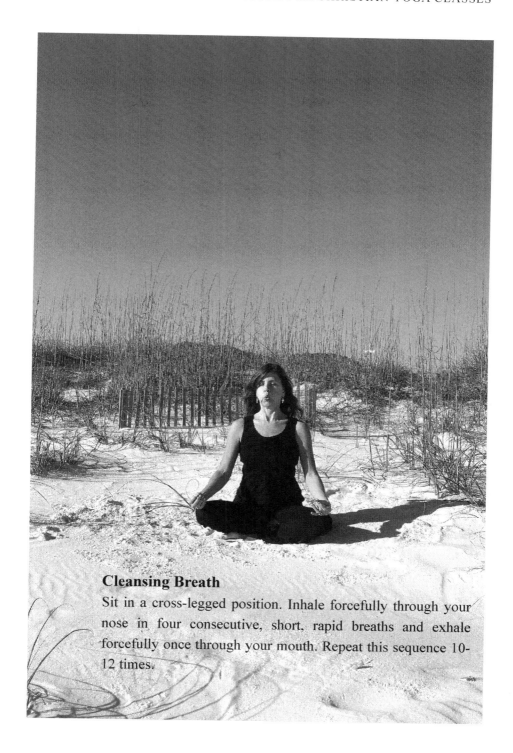

**Cleansing Breath**

Sit in a cross-legged position. Inhale forcefully through your nose in four consecutive, short, rapid breaths and exhale forcefully once through your mouth. Repeat this sequence 10-12 times.

## Squat

Place feet mat width apart and turn toes outward. Bend your knees, sink your tailbone down until it is lower than your knees. Wedge your elbows between the inside of your knees, palms together in a prayer position. Neck is straight and in alignment with the spine. Breathe deeply and hold for 3-4 breaths.

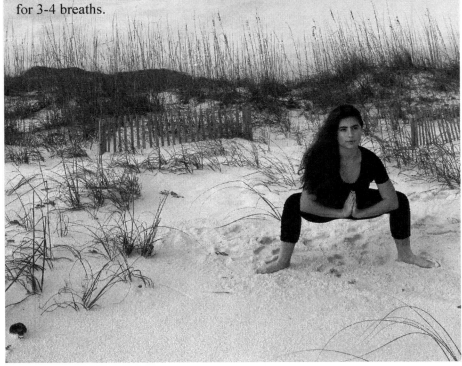

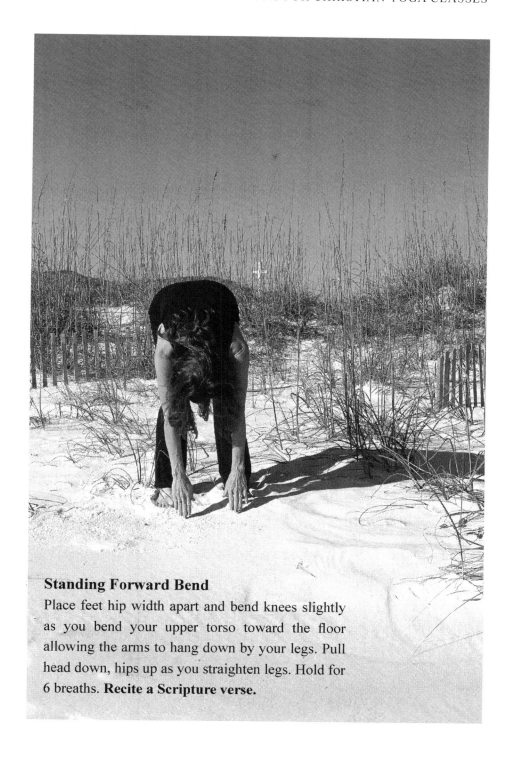

## Standing Forward Bend

Place feet hip width apart and bend knees slightly as you bend your upper torso toward the floor allowing the arms to hang down by your legs. Pull head down, hips up as you straighten legs. Hold for 6 breaths. **Recite a Scripture verse.**

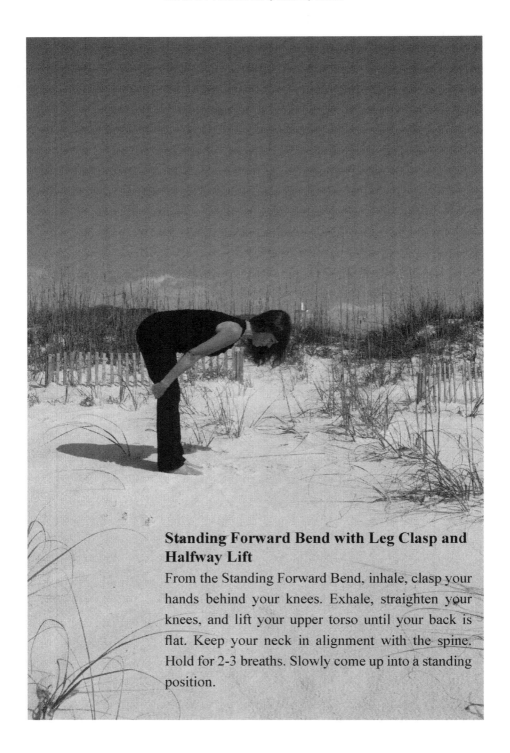

## Standing Forward Bend with Leg Clasp and Halfway Lift

From the Standing Forward Bend, inhale, clasp your hands behind your knees. Exhale, straighten your knees, and lift your upper torso until your back is flat. Keep your neck in alignment with the spine. Hold for 2-3 breaths. Slowly come up into a standing position.

## Standing Yoga Postures

Now we will begin our standing poses.

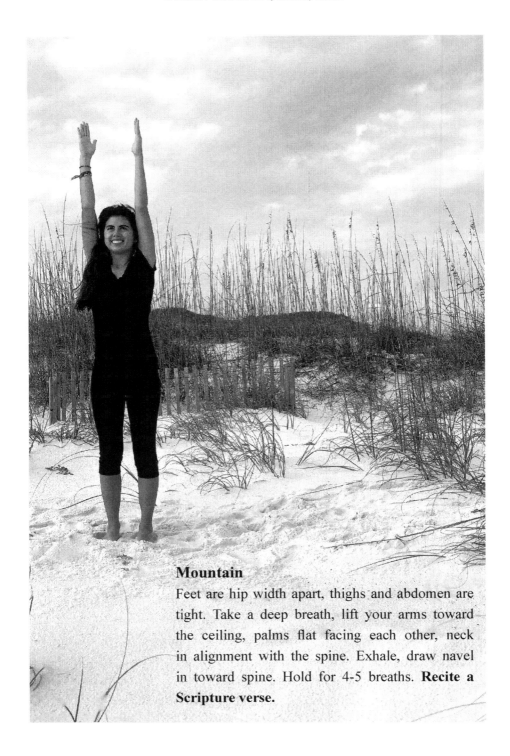

## Mountain

Feet are hip width apart, thighs and abdomen are tight. Take a deep breath, lift your arms toward the ceiling, palms flat facing each other, neck in alignment with the spine. Exhale, draw navel in toward spine. Hold for 4-5 breaths. **Recite a Scripture verse.**

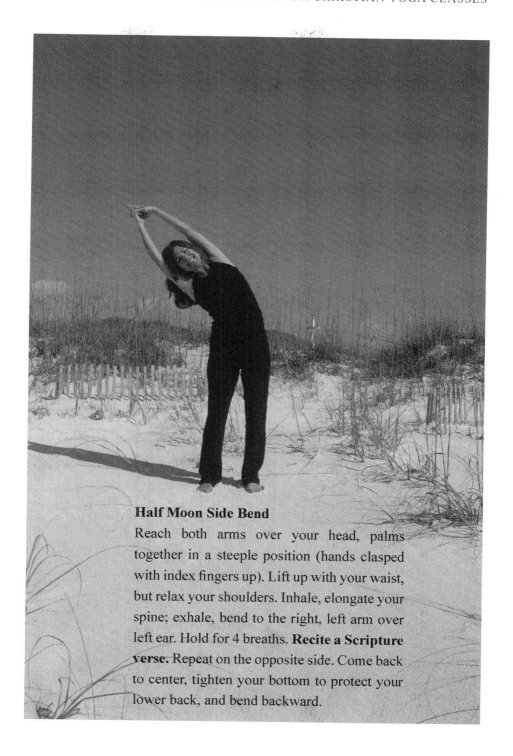

### Half Moon Side Bend

Reach both arms over your head, palms together in a steeple position (hands clasped with index fingers up). Lift up with your waist, but relax your shoulders. Inhale, elongate your spine; exhale, bend to the right, left arm over left ear. Hold for 4 breaths. **Recite a Scripture verse.** Repeat on the opposite side. Come back to center, tighten your bottom to protect your lower back, and bend backward.

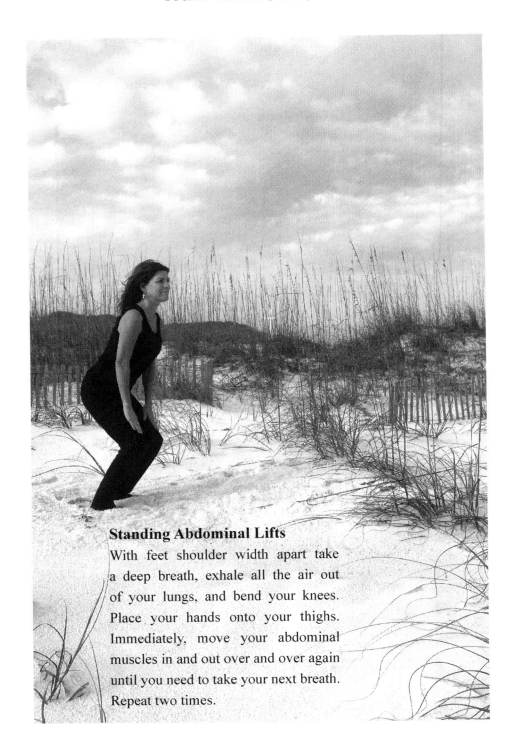

## Standing Abdominal Lifts

With feet shoulder width apart take a deep breath, exhale all the air out of your lungs, and bend your knees. Place your hands onto your thighs. Immediately, move your abdominal muscles in and out over and over again until you need to take your next breath. Repeat two times.

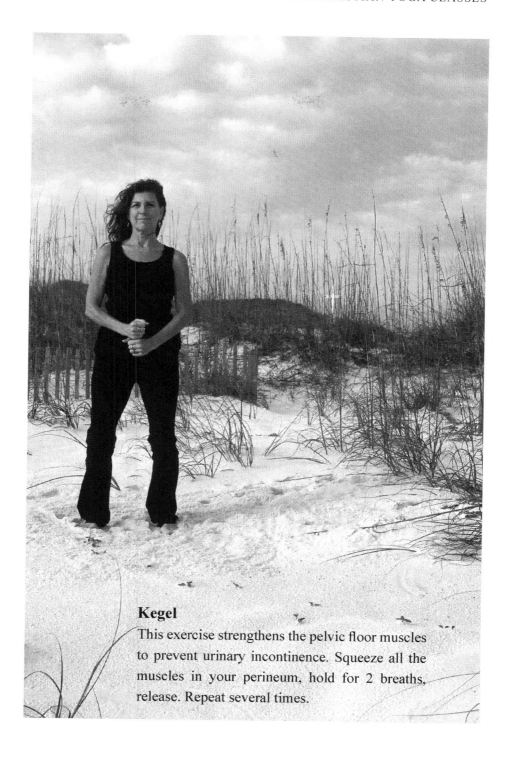

### Kegel

This exercise strengthens the pelvic floor muscles to prevent urinary incontinence. Squeeze all the muscles in your perineum, hold for 2 breaths, release. Repeat several times.

## Warrior I

Take a large step forward with your right foot. Make sure your right knee is over your ankle. Press the left heel toward the floor and keep this leg straight.

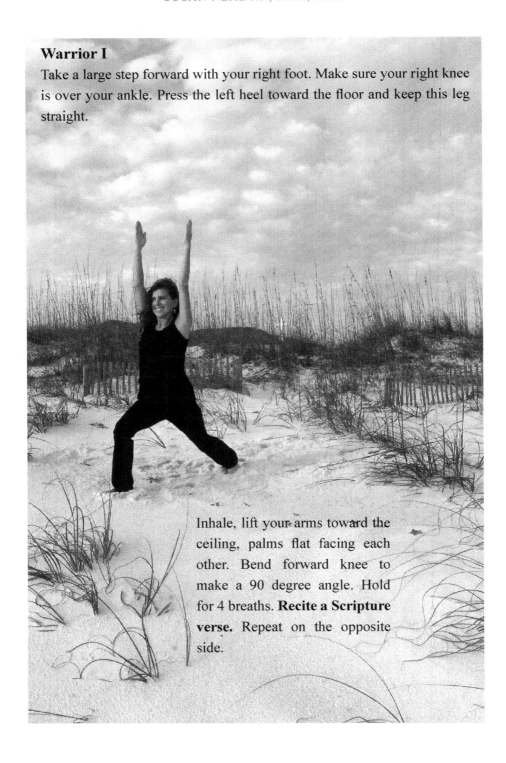

Inhale, lift your arms toward the ceiling, palms flat facing each other. Bend forward knee to make a 90 degree angle. Hold for 4 breaths. **Recite a Scripture verse.** Repeat on the opposite side.

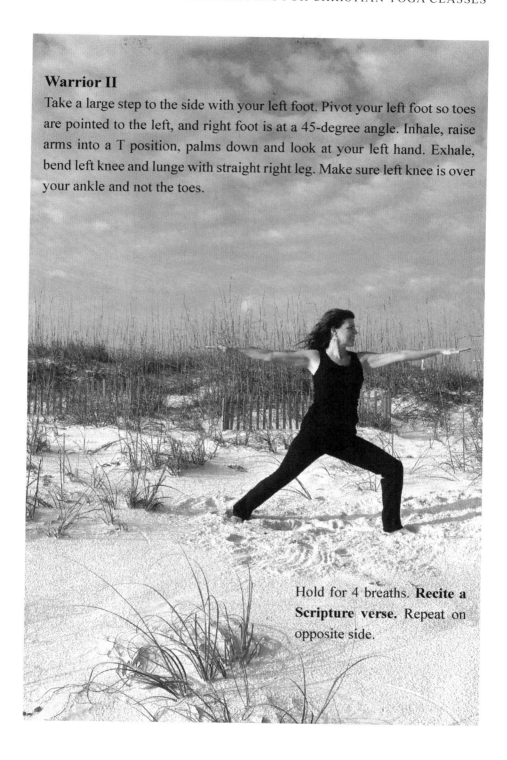

**Warrior II**

Take a large step to the side with your left foot. Pivot your left foot so toes are pointed to the left, and right foot is at a 45-degree angle. Inhale, raise arms into a T position, palms down and look at your left hand. Exhale, bend left knee and lunge with straight right leg. Make sure left knee is over your ankle and not the toes.

Hold for 4 breaths. **Recite a Scripture verse.** Repeat on opposite side.

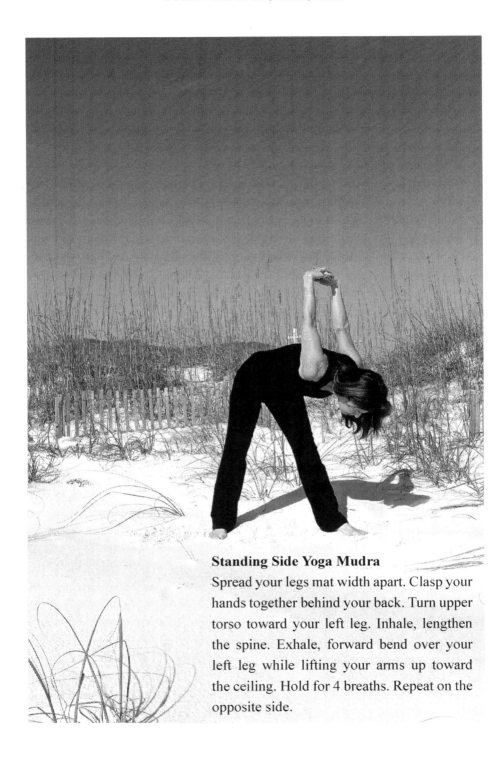

**Standing Side Yoga Mudra**

Spread your legs mat width apart. Clasp your hands together behind your back. Turn upper torso toward your left leg. Inhale, lengthen the spine. Exhale, forward bend over your left leg while lifting your arms up toward the ceiling. Hold for 4 breaths. Repeat on the opposite side.

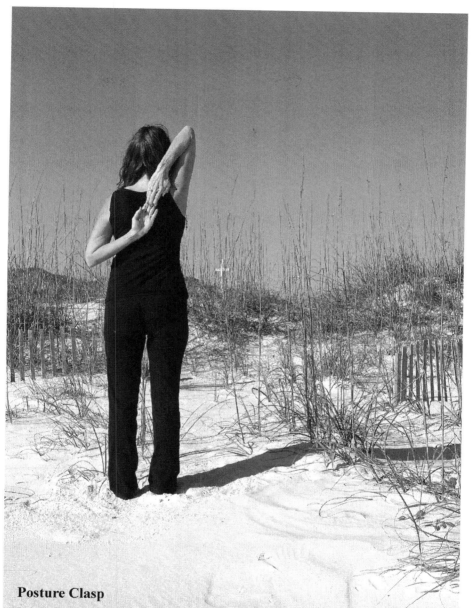

**Posture Clasp**

Inhale, lift your right hand over your head and reach for your right shoulder. Exhale, lower your left arm behind your back and reach for your right hand. Clasp your hands together, and move the left arm up and right down. Hold for 3-4 breaths. Repeat on the opposite side.

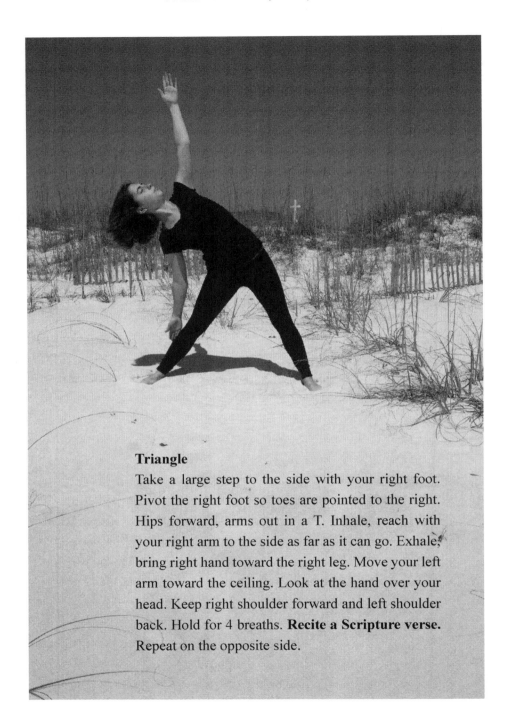

**Triangle**

Take a large step to the side with your right foot. Pivot the right foot so toes are pointed to the right. Hips forward, arms out in a T. Inhale, reach with your right arm to the side as far as it can go. Exhale, bring right hand toward the right leg. Move your left arm toward the ceiling. Look at the hand over your head. Keep right shoulder forward and left shoulder back. Hold for 4 breaths. **Recite a Scripture verse.** Repeat on the opposite side.

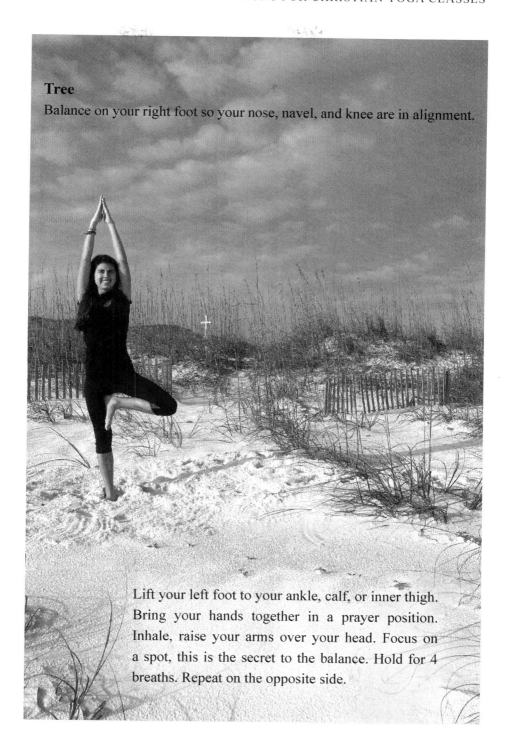

## Tree
Balance on your right foot so your nose, navel, and knee are in alignment.

Lift your left foot to your ankle, calf, or inner thigh. Bring your hands together in a prayer position. Inhale, raise your arms over your head. Focus on a spot, this is the secret to the balance. Hold for 4 breaths. Repeat on the opposite side.

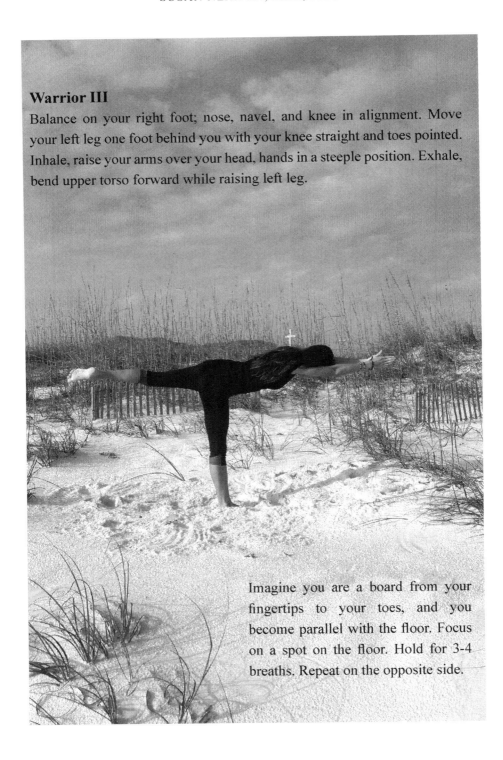

## Warrior III

Balance on your right foot; nose, navel, and knee in alignment. Move your left leg one foot behind you with your knee straight and toes pointed. Inhale, raise your arms over your head, hands in a steeple position. Exhale, bend upper torso forward while raising left leg.

Imagine you are a board from your fingertips to your toes, and you become parallel with the floor. Focus on a spot on the floor. Hold for 3-4 breaths. Repeat on the opposite side.

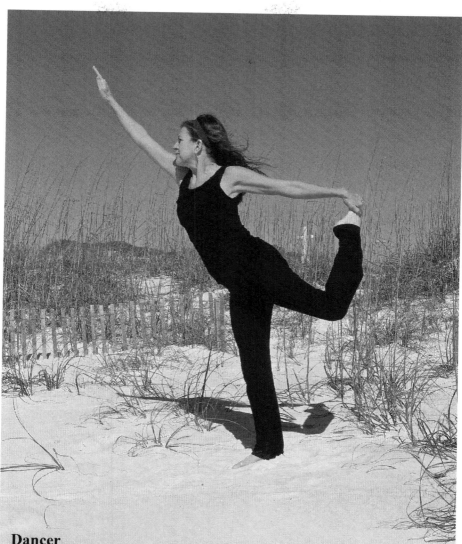

## Dancer

Balance on your right foot. Inhale, raise your right arm, elbow straight, over your head with fingertips pointed. Exhale, lift left foot behind you and grab it with your left hand. Lean forward with your upper body while pulling your left leg back behind you. Hold for 3-4 breaths. Repeat on the opposite side.

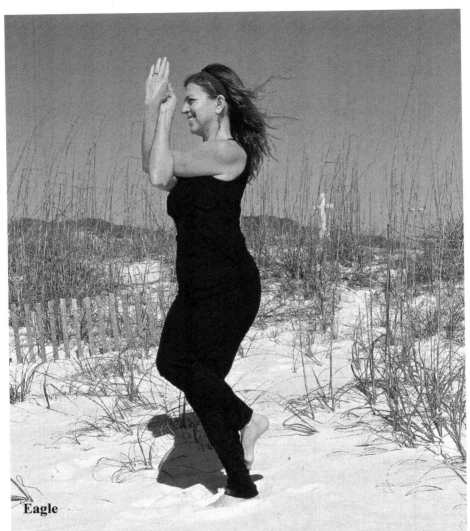

**Eagle**

Balance on your left foot and slightly bend the left knee. Cross your right thigh over your left thigh and wrap your right leg around the left. Hook right foot onto inside of left calf or ankle. Extend your left arm straight in front of you and cross right arm under the left. Bend your elbows and raise forearms perpendicular to the floor. Wrap forearms around each other with palms together in a prayer position, fingertips toward ceiling. Crown of head is pointed toward ceiling. Hold for 3-4 breaths.

## Prone or Belly Down Yoga Postures

Now that we have completed our standing postures we will lie down onto our bellies for our belly down poses.

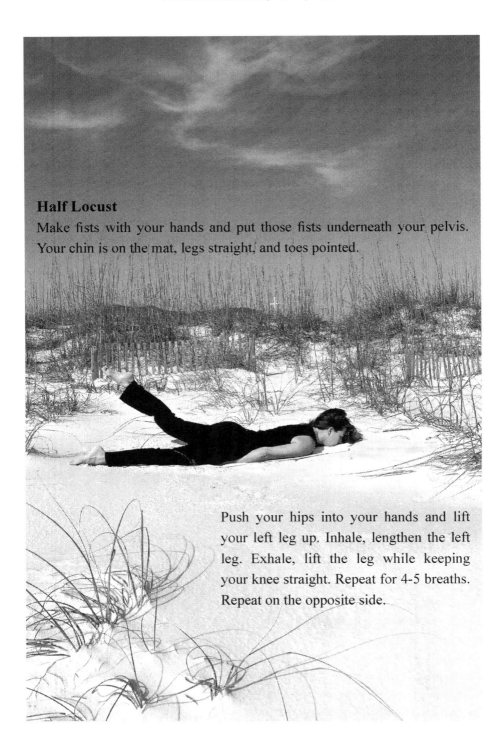

## Half Locust

Make fists with your hands and put those fists underneath your pelvis. Your chin is on the mat, legs straight, and toes pointed.

Push your hips into your hands and lift your left leg up. Inhale, lengthen the left leg. Exhale, lift the leg while keeping your knee straight. Repeat for 4-5 breaths. Repeat on the opposite side.

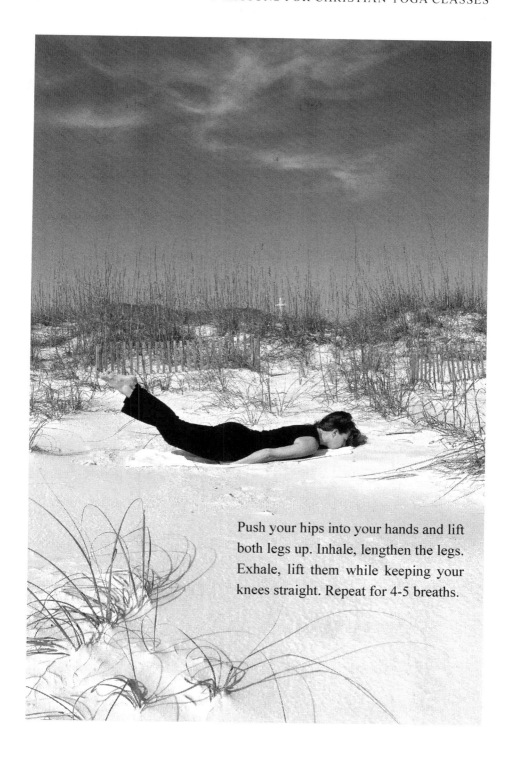

Push your hips into your hands and lift both legs up. Inhale, lengthen the legs. Exhale, lift them while keeping your knees straight. Repeat for 4-5 breaths.

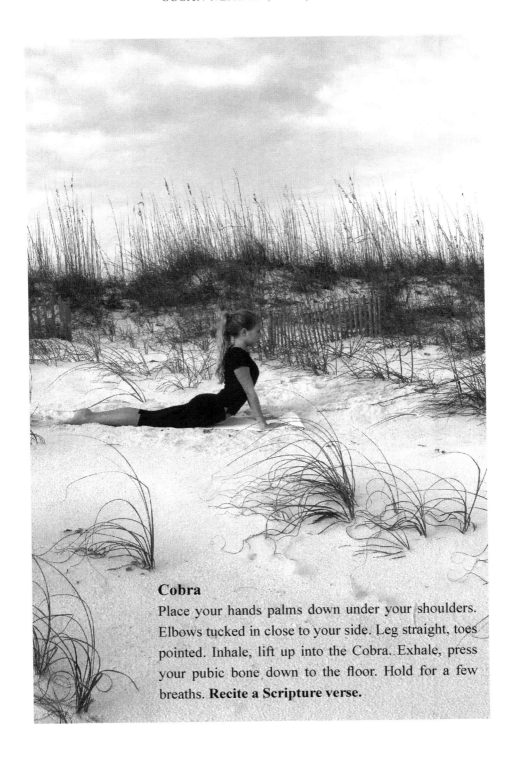

### Cobra

Place your hands palms down under your shoulders. Elbows tucked in close to your side. Leg straight, toes pointed. Inhale, lift up into the Cobra. Exhale, press your pubic bone down to the floor. Hold for a few breaths. **Recite a Scripture verse.**

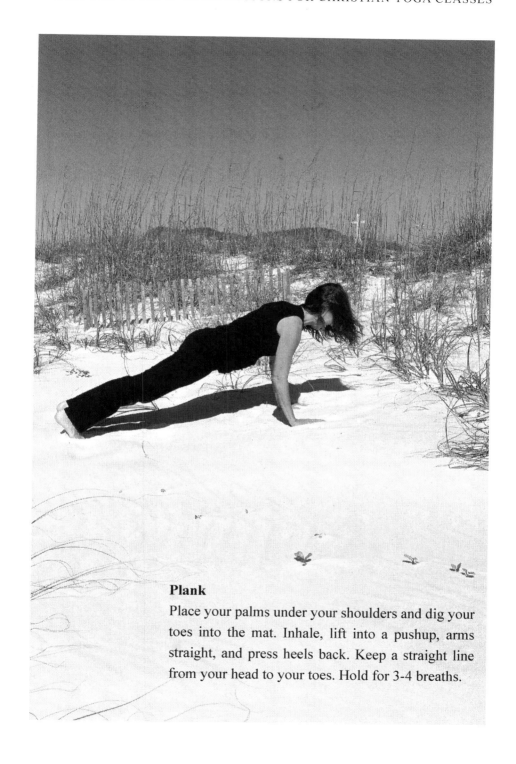

**Plank**

Place your palms under your shoulders and dig your toes into the mat. Inhale, lift into a pushup, arms straight, and press heels back. Keep a straight line from your head to your toes. Hold for 3-4 breaths.

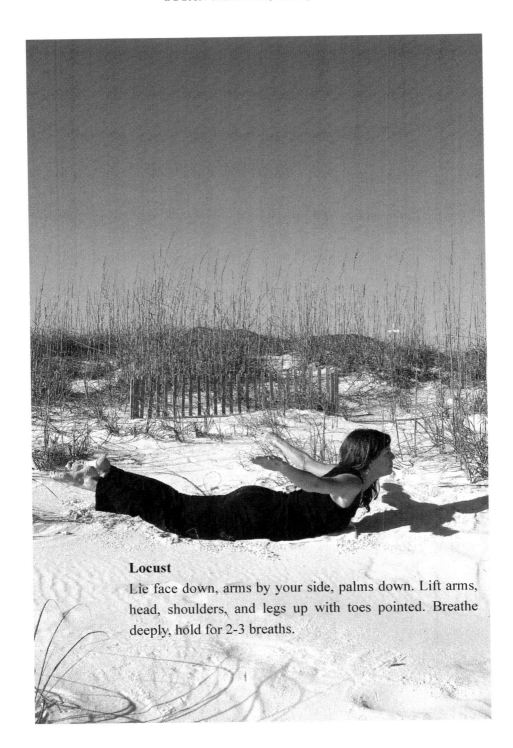

**Locust**
Lie face down, arms by your side, palms down. Lift arms, head, shoulders, and legs up with toes pointed. Breathe deeply, hold for 2-3 breaths.

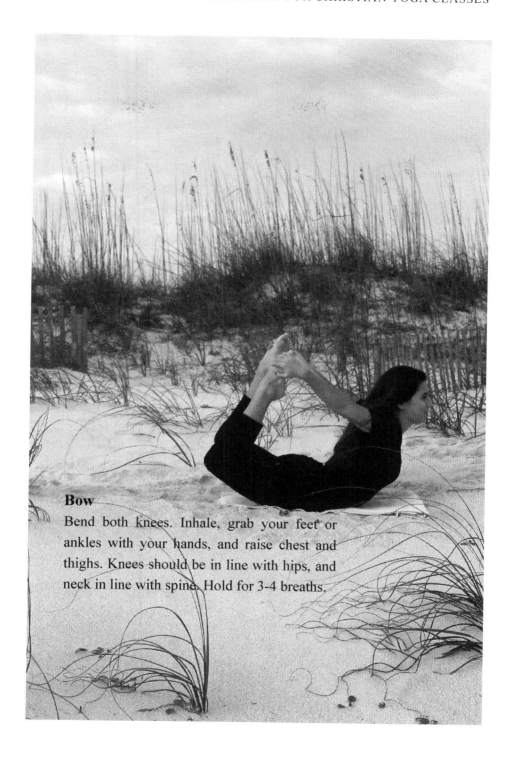

**Bow**
Bend both knees. Inhale, grab your feet or ankles with your hands, and raise chest and thighs. Knees should be in line with hips, and neck in line with spine. Hold for 3-4 breaths.

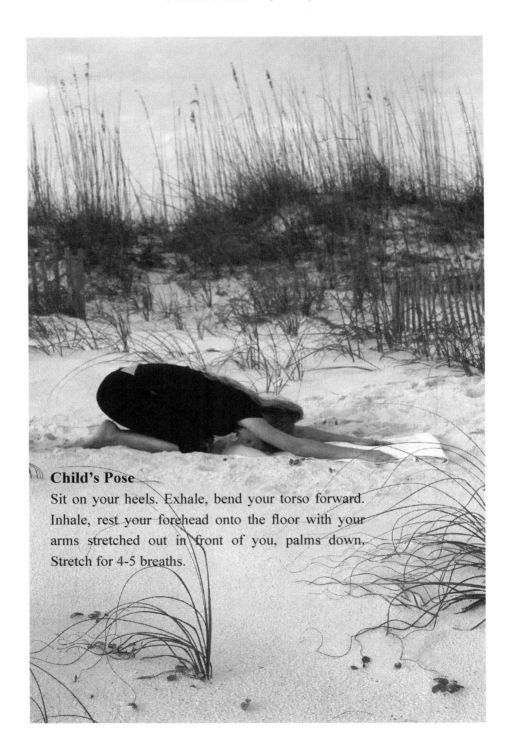

### Child's Pose

Sit on your heels. Exhale, bend your torso forward. Inhale, rest your forehead onto the floor with your arms stretched out in front of you, palms down. Stretch for 4-5 breaths.

## Supine or Back Down Yoga Postures

Get up and lie down onto your back for our back down postures.

**Double Leg Raises**

Lie on your back with your arms by your side. Raise both legs toward the ceiling. Keep your knees straight and buttocks on the mat. Slowly, lower your legs toward the floor and at the same time push your lower back down toward the floor.

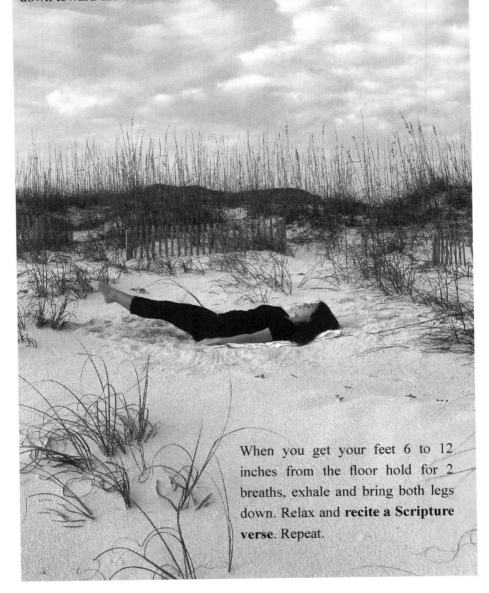

When you get your feet 6 to 12 inches from the floor hold for 2 breaths, exhale and bring both legs down. Relax and **recite a Scripture verse**. Repeat.

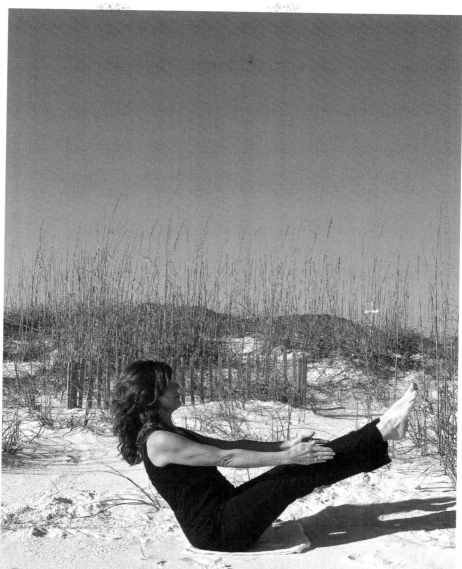

**Boat**

From a seated position, inhale, bend the knees; exhale, lift both legs up. Lean back, keep your neck in alignment with the spine. Straighten your legs and balance on your sits bone. Lift arms, elbows straight, so hands are by your knees. Hold for 3-4 breaths.

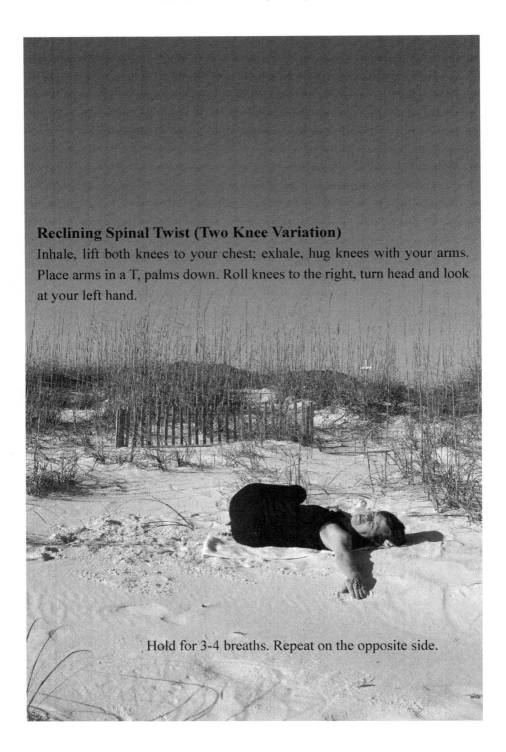

**Reclining Spinal Twist (Two Knee Variation)**
Inhale, lift both knees to your chest; exhale, hug knees with your arms.
Place arms in a T, palms down. Roll knees to the right, turn head and look
at your left hand.

Hold for 3-4 breaths. Repeat on the opposite side.

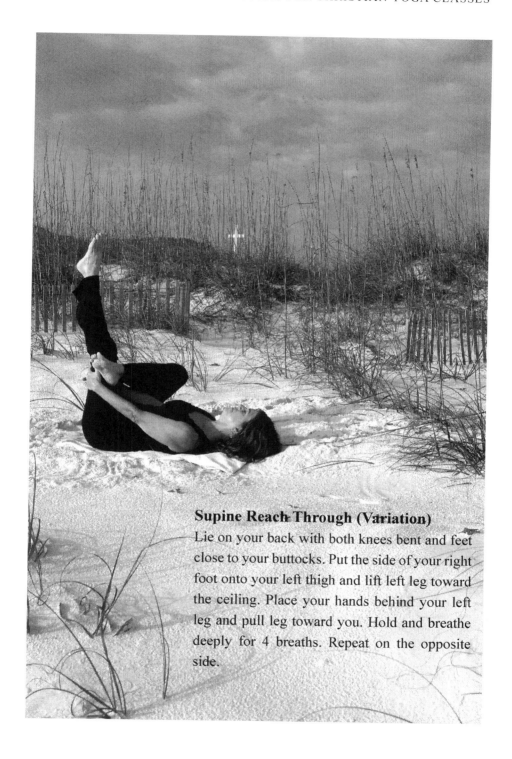

**Supine Reach Through (Variation)**
Lie on your back with both knees bent and feet close to your buttocks. Put the side of your right foot onto your left thigh and lift left leg toward the ceiling. Place your hands behind your left leg and pull leg toward you. Hold and breathe deeply for 4 breaths. Repeat on the opposite side.

## Bridge

Lie on your back with knees bent, feet close to your buttocks, and arms by your side, so fingertips touch heels. Inhale, firmly press feet into the mat. Exhale, lift your pelvis toward the ceiling so you are a straight line between your chest and pelvis. Distribute weight evenly between feet and shoulders. This is the basic posture of the bridge.

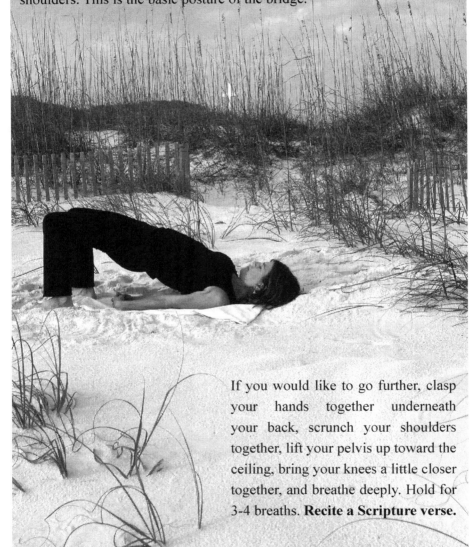

If you would like to go further, clasp your hands together underneath your back, scrunch your shoulders together, lift your pelvis up toward the ceiling, bring your knees a little closer together, and breathe deeply. Hold for 3-4 breaths. **Recite a Scripture verse.**

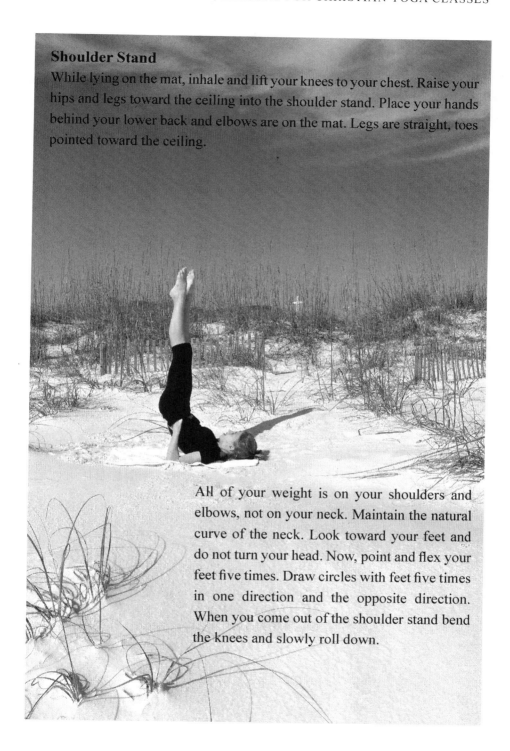

## Shoulder Stand

While lying on the mat, inhale and lift your knees to your chest. Raise your hips and legs toward the ceiling into the shoulder stand. Place your hands behind your lower back and elbows are on the mat. Legs are straight, toes pointed toward the ceiling.

All of your weight is on your shoulders and elbows, not on your neck. Maintain the natural curve of the neck. Look toward your feet and do not turn your head. Now, point and flex your feet five times. Draw circles with feet five times in one direction and the opposite direction. When you come out of the shoulder stand bend the knees and slowly roll down.

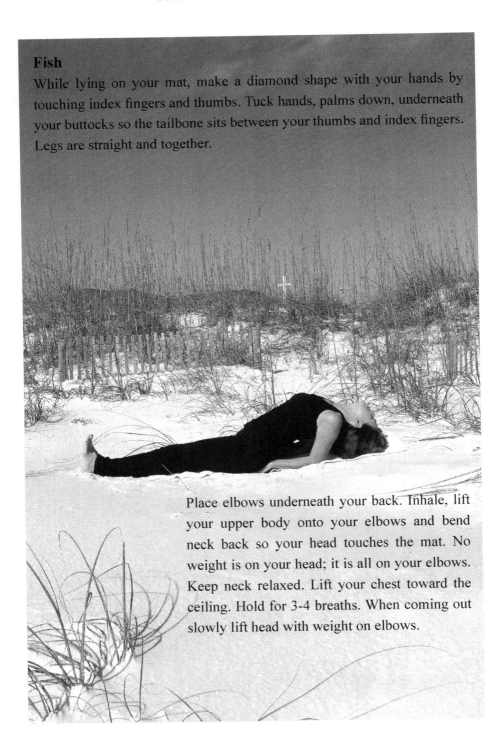

**Fish**

While lying on your mat, make a diamond shape with your hands by touching index fingers and thumbs. Tuck hands, palms down, underneath your buttocks so the tailbone sits between your thumbs and index fingers. Legs are straight and together.

Place elbows underneath your back. Inhale, lift your upper body onto your elbows and bend neck back so your head touches the mat. No weight is on your head; it is all on your elbows. Keep neck relaxed. Lift your chest toward the ceiling. Hold for 3-4 breaths. When coming out slowly lift head with weight on elbows.

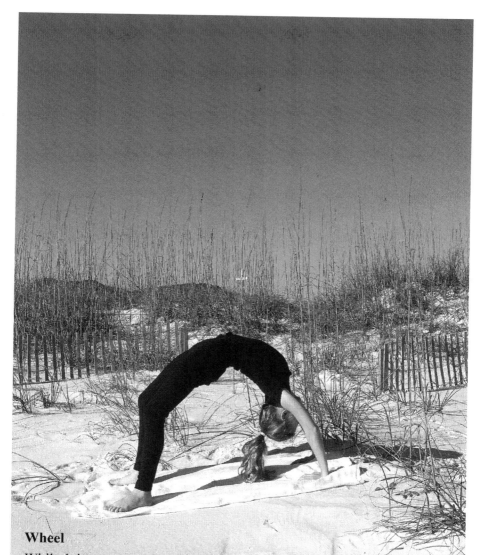

## Wheel

While lying on your back move your feet close to your buttocks. Place hands, palms down, onto the mat by your head with fingers pointed toward your toes. Inhale, firmly press your feet into the mat. Exhale, lift pelvis and abdomen toward the ceiling. Press heels down and engage legs. When coming down, bend your elbows and gently lie your head on the mat.

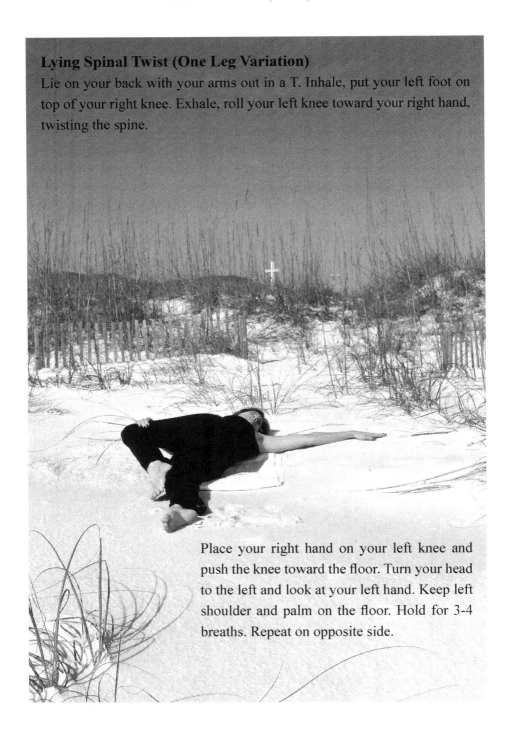

**Lying Spinal Twist (One Leg Variation)**

Lie on your back with your arms out in a T. Inhale, put your left foot on top of your right knee. Exhale, roll your left knee toward your right hand, twisting the spine.

Place your right hand on your left knee and push the knee toward the floor. Turn your head to the left and look at your left hand. Keep left shoulder and palm on the floor. Hold for 3-4 breaths. Repeat on opposite side.

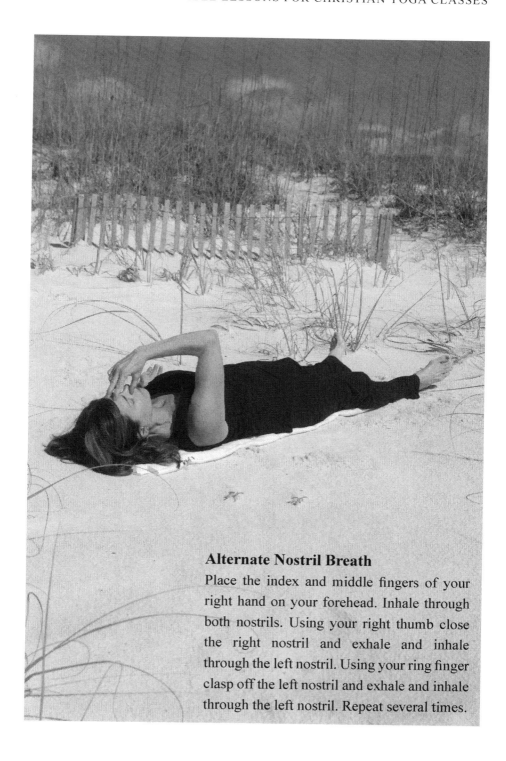

### Alternate Nostril Breath

Place the index and middle fingers of your right hand on your forehead. Inhale through both nostrils. Using your right thumb close the right nostril and exhale and inhale through the left nostril. Using your ring finger clasp off the left nostril and exhale and inhale through the left nostril. Repeat several times.

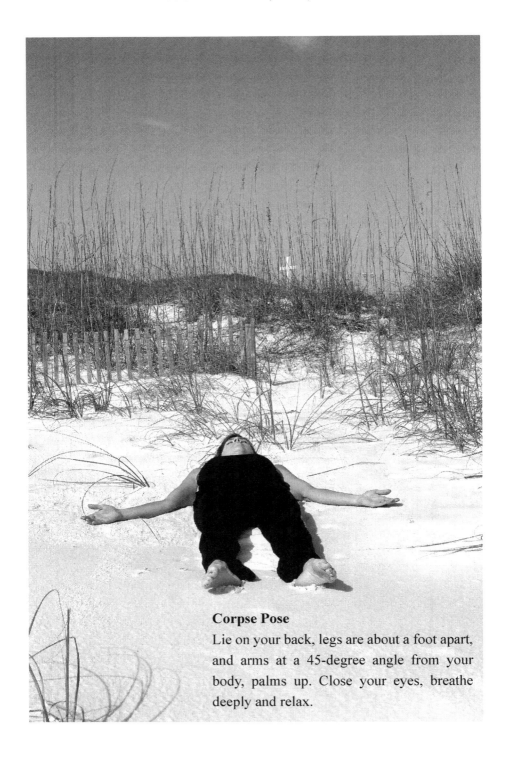

**Corpse Pose**

Lie on your back, legs are about a foot apart, and arms at a 45-degree angle from your body, palms up. Close your eyes, breathe deeply and relax.

You are going to relax your entire body from your head to your toes. Begin by relaxing your head. Relax each hair follicle from your forehead to the crown of your head, all the way down to the base of your neck.

Loosen your neck, shoulders, and shoulder blades. Relax the thoracic vertebra in the center of your back and all your muscles there. Relax your lumbar vertebra in your lower back and all those muscles. Relax your buttocks, sacrum, and tailbone. Your back is completely relaxed.

Now you will relax your face. Begin by releasing any tension in your forehead, eyes, and nose. Loosen your cheeks, ears, and jaw line all the way to your chin. Relax your lips. Swallow, relax your throat. Relax your neck from your chin all the way down your neck to your shoulders.

Release tension in your shoulders and upper arms all the way to your elbows. Relax your forearms, wrists, and hands. Allowing the tension to flow out through your fingertips.

Take a deep breath and know that your heart and lungs are functioning perfectly. Loosen your chest and abdominal muscles, all the way to your pelvis. Relax your intestinal organs, and the organs in your pelvis. Relax your pelvis.

Release the tension in your hips and thighs. The relaxation moves all the way down to the knees, calves, ankles, into the heels, up the feet, and out the toes.

Your body is completely at ease. You are lying in the palm of God's hand. You do not have a care in the world because you give all your cares to God.

**Recite a Scripture verse** — recite either the last verse in the lesson or the primary verse that you repeated throughout the class.

You are lying in the palm of God's hand, spend some time with him, and I will tell you when to get up in a few minutes.

Five minutes later: On the count of three you will become awake, alert, and energized. One, open your eyes and become aware of your surroundings. Two, wiggle your fingers and toes. Three, reach your arms over your head and stretch from your head to your toes.

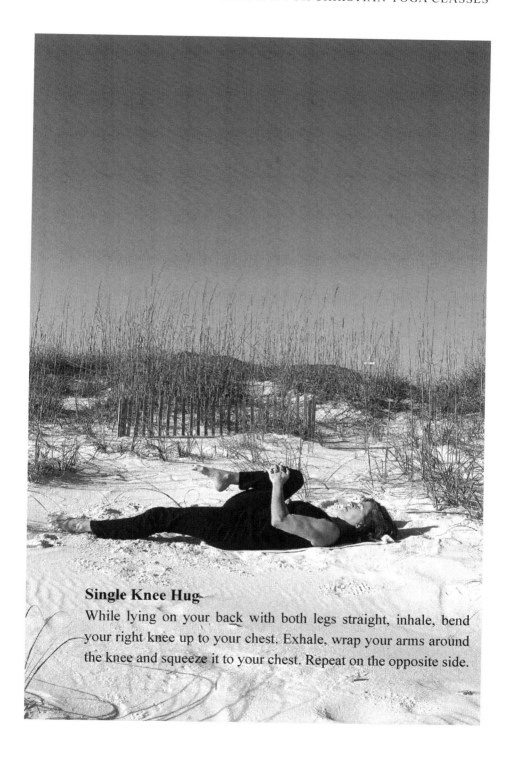

**Single Knee Hug**

While lying on your back with both legs straight, inhale, bend your right knee up to your chest. Exhale, wrap your arms around the knee and squeeze it to your chest. Repeat on the opposite side.

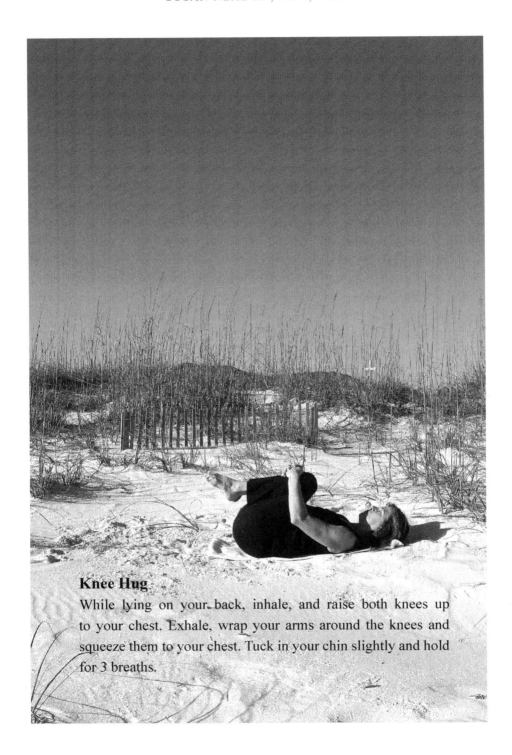

**Knee Hug**

While lying on your back, inhale, and raise both knees up to your chest. Exhale, wrap your arms around the knees and squeeze them to your chest. Tuck in your chin slightly and hold for 3 breaths.

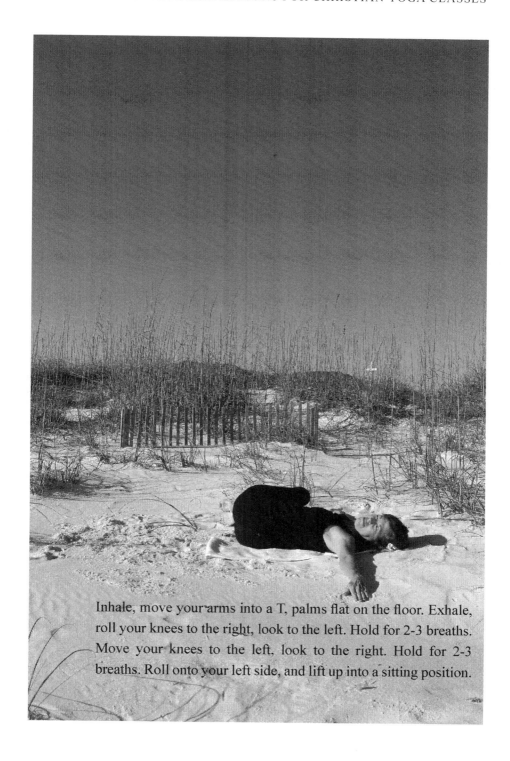

Inhale, move your arms into a T, palms flat on the floor. Exhale, roll your knees to the right, look to the left. Hold for 2-3 breaths. Move your knees to the left, look to the right. Hold for 2-3 breaths. Roll onto your left side, and lift up into a sitting position.

Scripture Yoga Cards with yoga poses and Scripture verses are available at ChristianYoga.com.

Please access the free Scripture Yoga class, "The Fall of Lucifer" at http://christianyoga.com/free. This is a brand new theme which is not included in this book. This Bible lesson answers the questions, "Why did Lucifer fall?" and "Why do bad things happen in this world?" You will also be notified when a deck of Scripture Yoga Cards become available.

# Chapter 5

# GOD'S GRACIOUS WORD

In each of the following Scripture theme chapters (Chapter 5-25), I use an * to differentiate between the Bible verse and my personal comment that I express to the class.

Matthew 4:4 (NIV)
Jesus answered, "It is written: 'Man shall not live on bread alone, but on every word that comes from the mouth of God.'"
*This verse is originally from Deuteronomy 8:3b. Jesus repeated it in Matthew 4:4.
Matthew 4:4 (The Message)
Jesus answered by quoting Deuteronomy: "It takes more than bread to stay alive. It takes a steady stream of words from God's mouth."

Acts 20:32 (The Message)
Now I'm turning you over to God, our marvelous God whose gracious Word can make you into what he wants you to be and give you everything you could possibly need in this community of holy friends.
*I repeat this verse, as the Holy Spirit leads me, several times during the class. This incorporates a central theme into the class.

John 1:1, 4 (NIV) *The Word Became Flesh*
In the beginning was the Word, and the Word was with God, and the Word was God. In him was life, and that life was the light of all mankind.

2 Corinthians 5:15 (LB)
He died for all so that who live — having received eternal life from him — might no longer live for themselves, to please themselves, but to spend their lives pleasing Christ who died and rose again for them.

Hebrews 4:12 (GW)
God's word is living and active. It is sharper than any two-edged sword and cuts as deep as the place where soul and spirit meet, the place where joints and marrow meet. God's word judges a person's thoughts and intentions.

2 Timothy 3:16
All Scripture is inspired by God and is useful to teach us what is true and to make us realize what is wrong in our lives. It corrects us when we are wrong and teaches us to do what is right.

Proverbs 2:6
For the LORD grants wisdom! From his mouth come knowledge and understanding.
*Sometimes I repeat this verse several times throughout the class. It is important for people to realize that we get knowledge, understanding, and wisdom from Scripture.

John 17:17
"Make them holy by your truth; teach them your word, which is truth."

John 17:17 (NCV)
"Make them ready for your service through your truth; your teaching is truth."

Colossians 3:10
Put on your new nature, and be renewed as you learn to know your Creator and become like him.

John 7:38 (LB)
"For the Scriptures declare rivers of living water shall flow from the inmost being of anyone who believes in me."

Proverbs 3:1–2 *Trusting in the LORD*
My child, never forget the things I have taught you. Store my commands in your heart. If you do this, you will live many years, and your life will be satisfying.

Joshua 1:8
Study this Book of Instruction continually. Meditate on it day and night so you will be sure to obey everything written in it. Only then will you prosper and succeed in all you do.

*I like to state the following verse when we are in the Mountain pose.
Psalm 1:1–3
Oh, the joys of those who do not follow the advice of the wicked, or stand around with sinners, or join in with mockers. But they delight in the law of the LORD, meditating on it day and night. They are like trees planted along the riverbank, bearing fruit each season. Their leaves never wither, and they prosper in all they do.

Psalm 107:20 (NIV)
He sent out his word and healed them; he rescued them from the grave.
*Sometimes I ask the class if they think God meant this literally (healing sickness) or figuratively (through sending us Jesus Christ).

Isaiah 55:10–11
The rain and snow come down from the heavens and stay on the ground to water the earth. They cause the grain to grow, producing seed for the farmer and bread for the hungry. It is the same with my word. I send it out, and it always produces fruit. It will accomplish all I want it to, and it will prosper everywhere I send it.

Luke 21:33 (NIV)

"Heaven and earth will pass away, but my words will never pass away."

*I tell the class that I am amazed by what this verse proclaims.

1 John 2:17 (NIV)

The world and its desires pass away, but whoever does the will of God lives forever.

*Author's notes

## Chapter 6

# THE FRUIT OF THE SPIRIT

Galatians 5:22–23

But the Holy Spirit produces this kind of fruit in our lives: love, joy, peace, patience, kindness, goodness, faithfulness, gentleness, and self-control. There is no law against these things!

*Anyone filled with the Holy Spirit is going to manifest these nine characteristics.

*The first fruit of the Spirit is Love: a love for God and fellow man. This is a love that causes someone to be more interested in the Kingdom of God rather than the material world.

Matthew 22:37

Jesus replied, "'You must love the LORD your God with all your heart, all your soul, and all your mind.' "

Matthew 19:19b (NIV)

"love your neighbor as yourself."

Matthew 5:44 (KJV 1900)

"But I say unto you, Love your enemies, bless them that curse you, do good to them that hate you, and pray for them which despitefully use you, and persecute you;"

John 13:35

"Your love for one another will prove to the world that you are my disciples."

*The second fruit of the Spirit is joy! It is an enduring joy that bubbles up from the grace of God. Circumstances do not limit the joy provided by the Holy Spirit.

John 15:10–11

"When you obey my commandments, you remain in my love, just as I obey my Father's commandments and remain in his love. I have told you these things so that you will be filled with my joy. Yes, your joy will overflow!"

Philippians 4:11 b (NRSV)

for I have learned to be content with whatever I have.

*The third fruit of the Spirit is Peace. Peace from God is the peace of an untroubled heart.

John 14:27

"I am leaving you with a gift—peace of mind and heart. And the peace I give is a gift the world cannot give."

Philippians 4:6–7

Don't worry about anything; instead, pray about everything. Tell God what you need, and thank him for all he has done. Then you will experience God's peace, which exceeds anything we can understand. His peace will guard your hearts and minds as you live in Christ Jesus.

*The fourth fruit of the Spirit is patience, also called longsuffering or endurance. This involves the ability to bear insults without answering in the same way.

Proverbs 15:1

A gentle answer deflects anger, but harsh words make tempers flare.

1 Peter 2:23

He did not retaliate when he was insulted, nor threaten revenge when he suffered.

*A patient person is one who can do the menial tasks of life without complaining or brooding.

*The fifth fruit of the Spirit is kindness, which flows from an unselfish heart. Kindness is being gracious to others, especially in dealing with their faults.

Ephesians 4:32

Instead, be kind to each other, tenderhearted, forgiving one another, just as God through Christ has forgiven you.

*Goodness is the sixth fruit of the Spirit. It is generous with self and possessions. It is benevolence and hospitality.

Acts 20:35

And I have been a constant example of how you can help those in need by working hard. You should remember the words of the Lord Jesus: 'It is more blessed to give than to receive.'

1 Timothy 6:18

Tell them to use their money to do good. They should be rich in good works and generous to those in need, always being ready to share with others.

*The seventh fruit of the Spirit is faith, which involves the complete abandonment of yourself and your life to God. It is a dependence upon him. Faith is the perfect antidote to fear, which causes worry and anxiety.

Romans 10:17 (ESV)

So faith comes from hearing, and hearing through the word of Christ.

*Therefore, to increase your faith you need to read the Word of God.

*Gentleness is the eighth fruit of the Spirit. It is the tenderheartedness behind a thoughtful, considerate act of kindness.
James 3:17
But the wisdom from above is first of all pure. It is also peace loving, gentle at all times, and willing to yield to others.

Proverbs 15:4
Gentle words are a tree of life;

*The ninth fruit of the Spirit is self-control. This is the reigning in of any emotional excesses.
Proverbs 16:32
Better to have self-control than to conquer a city.

2 Timothy 1:7 (RSV)
for God did not give us a spirit of timidity but a spirit of power and love and self-control.

*The Spirit controlled temperament will be consistent, dependable, and well-ordered.

*The teaching for this class was inspired by a book by Tim LaHaye titled *"Spirit-Controlled Temperament"* (1994).

*Author's notes

The author has published a deck of Scripture Yoga Cards: "Fruit of the Spirit." You can find the cards at: http://christianyoga.com/yoga-books-decks.

## Chapter 7

# THE GREATEST GIFT OF THEM ALL–LOVE

Ephesians 3:18
And may you have the power to understand, as all God's people should, how wide, how long, how high, and how deep his love is.
*Try to understand how much God loves YOU!

1 John 4:16b
God is love, and all who live in love live in God, and God lives in them.
*Now think of this verse as three bowls: large, medium, and small. God is the large bowl, you are the medium bowl that fits inside God's love, and the Holy Spirit is the small bowl that fits inside of you.

2 Corinthians 5: 21 (LB)
For God took the sinless Christ and poured into him our sins. Then, in exchange, he poured God's goodness into us!
*I saw this as an example at a Loving Well Retreat in a Box by Beth Moore. Three glasses filled with water represented Jesus, us, and God. The first crystal clear glass symbolized Christ. Beth poured a glass filled with muddy water, which represented our sins, into Jesus' glass. Then she poured a liquid from God's glass into our muddy sinful water, and the liquid from God made our muddy water crystal clear (Moore, 2005). After explaining this, re-read the Scripture above so your yoga class participants can visualize the example.

Hebrews 10:9–10 (NCV)

God ends the first system of sacrifices so he can set up the new system. And because of this, we are made holy through the sacrifice Christ made in his body once and for all time.

John 13:34–35

"So now I am giving you a new commandment: Love each other. Just as I have loved you, you should love each other. Your love for one another will prove to the world that you are my disciples."

Matthew 5:44–45a

"But I say, love your enemies! Pray for those who persecute you! In that way, you will be acting as true children of your Father in heaven."

1 John 3:16–19a

We know what real love is because Jesus gave up his life for us. So we also ought to give up our lives for our brothers and sisters. If someone has enough money to live well and sees a brother or sister in need but shows no compassion—how can God's love be in that person? Dear children, let's not merely say that we love each other; let us show the truth by our actions. Our actions will show that we belong to the truth,

*And what is the truth?

John 14:6

Jesus told him, "I am the way, the truth, and the life. No one can come to the Father except through me."

1 John 4:9–10

God showed how much he loved us by sending his one and only Son into the world so that we might have eternal life through him. This is real love—not that we loved God, but that he loved us and sent his Son as a sacrifice to take away our sins.

1 Corinthians 13:4a
Love is patient and kind.

1 Corinthians 14:1a
Let love be your highest goal!

Proverbs 15:1
A gentle answer deflects anger, but harsh words make tempers flare.

1 Peter 3:9
Don't repay evil for evil. Don't retaliate with insults when people insult you. Instead, pay them back with a blessing. That is what God has called you to do, and he will bless you for it.

1 Corinthians 13:7
Love never gives up, never loses faith, is always hopeful, and endures through every circumstance.

1 John 4:16b (NIV)
God is love.


*Author's notes

# Chapter 8

# HOW TO BE FILLED WITH THE HOLY SPIRIT

This theme was inspired by the book *Spirit-Controlled Temperament* by Tim LaHaye (1994). Tim indicates there are five steps to be filled with the Holy Spirit.

1. Examine yourself for sin.

1 Corinthians 11:31 (NRSV)
But if we judged ourselves, we would not be judged.

1 Corinthians 11:28
you should examine yourself before eating the bread and drinking the cup.
*Ask the class to take a moment to examine their own heart for sin.

*We cannot be filled with sin and the Holy Spirit at the same time. So you need to complete the second step to be filled with the Spirit which is:

2. Confess your sins to God.

1 John 1:9
But if we confess our sins to him, he is faithful and just to forgive us our sins and to cleanse us from all wickedness.
*Let us each take a moment to confess our sins to God.

3. Submit yourself completely to God.

James 4:7 (ISV)
Therefore, submit yourselves to God. Resist the devil, and he will run away from you.

Psalm 2:12
Submit to God's royal son,

4. Ask God to fill you with His Spirit.

5. To walk in the Spirit means to abide in Christ.
*What is abiding in Christ? To me, it is having God be present with me throughout the day. At any moment, I can speak with him or call upon him. It is being aware of his presence just like you would be if you were pregnant.

Galatians 5:16
Let the Holy Spirit guide your lives. Then you won't be doing what your sinful nature craves.

Galatians 5:25
Since we are living by the Spirit, let us follow the Spirit's leading in every part of our lives.
*I explain how it is important to listen to the small, quiet voice inside of us, which is the Holy Spirit.

*Tim LaHaye (1994) states that being filled with the Holy Spirit is not a single experience but must be repeated many times.
*I repeat the five steps: Examine yourself for sin, repent, submit yourself to God, ask to be filled with the Holy Spirit, and walk in the Spirit.

*Walking in the Spirit needs a daily feeding on the Word of God. So open your Bible and read it every day, even if it is only one verse.

*Author's notes

# Chapter 9

# DON'T QUENCH THE SPIRIT

Two destructive emotions that quench the Holy Spirit are anger and fear. This theme is from the book, *Spirit Controlled Temperament,* by Tim LaHaye (1994).

*Most people have a tendency toward being either angry or fearful. Which are you?

*Here are a couple verses regarding anger.
Ephesians 4:26
And "don't sin by letting anger control you."

*In a different version of the Bible this same verse (Ephesians 4:26 ESV) states:
"Be angry and do not sin;"

Ephesians 4:27
for anger gives a foothold to the devil.

*The second emotion that quenches the Spirit is fear.
Matthew 6:25, 27
"That is why I tell you not to worry about everyday life—whether you have enough food and drink, or enough clothes to wear. Isn't life more than food, and your body more than clothing? Can all your worries add a single moment to your life?"

1 Peter 5:7
Give all your worries and cares to God, for he cares about you.

*The following is the same verse, but from a different version of the Bible.
1 Peter 5:7 (NIV)
Cast all your anxiety on him because he cares for you.
*In this verse, cast means to hurl or throw. Therefore, you have to choose to give God your anxiety and worries.

*Anger and fear can be traced to sins of selfishness.

*Two causes of selfishness are:
1. Egotism—This is the root of anger
2. Low self-esteem—which is the source of fear

*During the class, I humbly admit what my problem is: anger and egotism. Admit yours.

Philippians 2:3–4
Don't be selfish; don't try to impress others. Be humble, thinking of others as better than yourselves. Don't look out only for your own interests, but take an interest in others, too.

*The good news is that you can overcome selfishness with God's help.

*When we surrender our life entirely to Jesus Christ, the Spirit of God will cure our problem of selfishness.

Matthew 10:39
"If you cling to your life, you will lose it; but if you give up your life for me, you will find it."

*What are you clinging to in your life?

Luke 8:15
"And the seeds that fell on the good soil represent honest, good-hearted people who hear God's word, cling to it, and patiently produce a huge harvest."

*Now, I pray for the class: Lord, please help our hearts to be the good soil that the word of God is planted in and help us to produce a huge harvest for you.

Proverbs 2:6 (NIV)
For the LORD gives wisdom; from his mouth come knowledge and understanding.

*Author's notes

# Chapter 10

# TEMPTATION AND
# THE EVIL ONE

*God did not accept Cain's grain offering, and this made Cain furious.
So God spoke to him:
Genesis 4:6–7
"Why are you so angry?" the LORD asked Cain. "Why do you look so
dejected? You will be accepted if you do what is right. But if you refuse
to do what is right, then watch out! Sin is crouching at the door, eager to
control you. But you must subdue it and be its master."

1 Corinthians 10:13b
And God is faithful. He will not allow the temptation to be more than
you can stand. When you are tempted, he will show you a way out so
that you can endure.

*Explain the following situation to the class (verses 31-32). Then recite
verse 33.
Mark 8:31a–33 *Jesus Predicts His Death*
Then Jesus began to tell them that the Son of Man must suffer many
terrible things and be rejected... He would be killed, but three days
later he would rise from the dead. ³² As he talked about this openly
with his disciples, Peter took him aside and began to reprimand him for
saying such things. ³³ Jesus turned around and looked at his disciples,
then reprimanded Peter. "Get away from me, Satan!" he said. "You are
seeing things merely from a human point of view, not from God's."

2 Corinthians 12:9

Each time he said, "My grace is all you need. My power works best in weakness." So now I am glad to boast about my weaknesses, so that the power of Christ can work through me.

*Tell the class "God does not call the equipped, he equips the called."

Matthew 6:13

"And don't let us yield to temptation, but rescue us from the evil one."

*I find it interesting that there are two parts to the following verse. Many times we hear only the second sentence of this verse. I believe that to resist the devil you must first submit yourself to God, just like this verse declares.

James 4:7 (ESV)

Submit yourselves therefore to God. Resist the devil, and he will flee from you.

1 John 4:4b (NCV)

because God's Spirit, who is in you, is greater than the devil, who is in the world.

Luke 10:19a

"Look, I have given you authority over all the power of the enemy,"

*This is the verse I use when casting Satan and his evil spirits out of my life. First, I confess my sins and then pray beginning with this verse.

*Jesus responded to Satan's temptation with Scripture. That is how we should fight Satan as well. If you struggle with a problem, find a verse to fight it. Write the verse down on an index card and use it against our enemy!

Matthew 4:10

"Get out of here, Satan," Jesus told him. "For the Scriptures say, 'You must worship the LORD your God and serve only him.'"

*For example, someone can fight the tendency to use alcohol or drugs with this verse.
Ephesians 5:18
Don't be drunk with wine, because that will ruin your life. Instead, be filled with the Holy Spirit,

John 10:10
"The thief's purpose is to steal and kill and destroy. My purpose is to give them a rich and satisfying life."

2 Corinthians 4:4a
Satan, who is the god of this world, has blinded the minds of those who don't believe. They are unable to see the glorious light of the Good News.

2 Corinthians 11:13a–14
These people are false apostles. But I am not surprised! Even Satan disguises himself as an angel of light.

Ephesians 4:26a–27
And "don't sin by letting anger control you." for anger gives a foothold to the devil.

*The following verse explains how unforgiveness and resentment opens a door into your life for Satan to begin his 'ugly small talk' in your brain.
2 Corinthians 2:11 (LB)
A further reason for forgiveness is to keep you from being outsmarted by Satan, for we know what he is trying to do.

Matthew 6:15
"But if you refuse to forgive others, your Father will not forgive your sins."

James 1:12a (ISV) *Our Desires Tempt Us*
How blessed is the man who endures temptation! When he has passed the test, he will receive the victor's crown of life that God has promised those who keep on loving him.


*Author's notes

## Chapter 11

# OUR ADVOCATE: THE HOLY SPIRIT

*A Pharisee named Nicodemus came to speak with Jesus, after dark, one evening and Jesus told him:

John 3:6b–8

"but the Holy Spirit gives birth to spiritual life. So don't be surprised when I say, 'You must be born again.' The wind blows wherever it wants. Just as you can hear the wind but can't tell where it comes from or where it is going, so you can't explain how people are born of the Spirit."

John 14:26

"But when the Father sends the Advocate as my representative—that is, the Holy Spirit—he will teach you everything and will remind you of everything I have told you."

John 15:26

"But I will send you the Advocate—the Spirit of truth. He will come to you from the Father and will testify all about me."

John 16:13a

"When the Spirit of truth comes, he will guide you into all truth."

John 16:8

"And when he comes, he will convict the world of its sin, and of God's righteousness, and of the coming judgment."

John 14:17

"He is the Holy Spirit, who leads into all truth. The world cannot receive him, because it isn't looking for him and doesn't recognize him. But you know him, because he lives with you now and later will be in you."

John 16:7

"But in fact, it is best for you that I go away, because if I don't, the Advocate won't come. If I do go away, then I will send him to you."
*Jesus had to die to fulfill his mission on earth: to defeat sin, Satan, and death before the Holy Spirit could come.

Acts 1:8a

"But you will receive power when the Holy Spirit comes upon you. And you will be my witnesses"
*All of the verses we have recited so far were stated by Jesus.

Acts 2:1–4a  *The Holy Spirit Comes*

On the day of Pentecost all the believers were meeting together in one place. Suddenly, there was a sound from heaven like the roaring of a mighty windstorm, and it filled the house where they were sitting. Then, what looked like flames or tongues of fire appeared and settled on each of them. And everyone present was filled with the Holy Spirit.

*All of the following verses were expressed by Paul.
2 Corinthians 3:18b

And the Lord—who is the Spirit—makes us more and more like him as we are changed into his glorious image.
*An ultimate goal in life should be to be more like Jesus!

Galatians 4:6a

And because we are his children, God has sent the Spirit of his Son into our hearts,"
The Spirit of his son is the Holy Spirit.

1 Corinthians 2:14 (GW)
A person who isn't spiritual doesn't accept the teachings of God's Spirit. He thinks they're nonsense. He can't understand them because a person must be spiritual to evaluate them.

1 Corinthians 2:16b (LB)
But strange as it seems, we Christians actually do have within us a portion of the very thoughts and mind of Christ.

1 Corinthians 6:19–20 (GW)
Don't you know that your body is a temple that belongs to the Holy Spirit? The Holy Spirit, whom you received from God, lives in you. You don't belong to yourselves. You were bought for a price. So bring glory to God in the way you use your body.

Romans 8:2
And because you belong to him, the power of the life-giving Spirit has freed you from the power of sin that leads to death.

Ephesians 1:13
And when you believed in Christ, he identified you as his own by giving you the Holy Spirit, whom he promised long ago.

Romans 8:10
And Christ lives within you, so even though your body will die because of sin, the Spirit gives you life because you have been made right with God.

Romans 8:11
The Spirit of God, who raised Jesus from the dead, lives in you. And just as God raised Christ Jesus from the dead, he will give life to your mortal bodies by this same Spirit living within you.

Romans 8:5b

but those who are controlled by the Holy Spirit think about things that please the Spirit.

Romans 8:9

But you are not controlled by your sinful nature. You are controlled by the Spirit if you have the Spirit of God living in you.

Romans 8:6b

But letting the Spirit control your mind leads to life and peace.

1 Corinthians 2:16b

But we understand these things, for we have the mind of Christ.

*Author's notes

# *Chapter 12*

# HOW TO RECEIVE GOD'S PEACE

This is one of my favorite themes. Everyone needs to learn how to give God their anxiety and fears and replace it with his peace, a peace the world cannot give us.

Psalms 23:1-3 (LB)
Because the Lord is my Shepherd, I have everything I need! He lets me rest in the meadow grass and leads me beside the quiet streams. He gives me new strength. He helps me do what honors him the most.

Isaiah 26:3
You will keep in perfect peace all who trust in you, all whose thoughts are fixed on you!
*If something is worrying me, I pray about it every time the thought enters my mind. This will give you God's perfect peace.

Psalm 50:15 (NIV)
"call on me in the day of trouble; I will deliver you, and you will honor me."
*Call upon God to help you whenever you experience trouble, and you will honor and glorify him.

Psalm 37:5
Commit everything you do to the LORD. Trust him, and he will help you.

1 Peter 5:7 (NIV)
Cast all your anxiety on him because he cares for you.
*In this verse, cast means to hurl or throw, like you would cast a fishing line.

*In the New Living Translation of the Bible the same verse reads:
1 Peter 5:7
Give all your worries and cares to God, for he cares about you.
*You have to choose to give God your burdens. You can keep them or cast them to the Lord.

2 Timothy 1:7
For God has not given us a spirit of fear and timidity, but of power, love, and self-discipline.
*We need to give our fears and insecurities to God too.

Isaiah 41:10
Don't be afraid, for I am with you. Don't be discouraged, for I am your God. I will strengthen you and help you. I will hold you up with my victorious right hand.

Philippians 4:6–7
Don't worry about anything; instead, pray about everything. Tell God what you need, and thank him for all he has done. Then you will experience God's peace, which exceeds anything we can understand. His peace will guard your hearts and minds as you live in Christ Jesus.
*I have put this important verse into a mathematical equation:
Don't Worry + Pray + Thank God + Abide in Christ = God's Peace

Psalm 46:1 (GW)
God is our refuge and strength, an ever-present help in times of trouble.
*When I have a serious situation going on in my life, I repeat this verse over and over again.

Matthew 11:28–30 (NIV)
"Come to me, all you who are weary and burdened, and I will give you rest. Take my yoke upon you and learn from me, for I am gentle and humble in heart, and you will find rest for your souls. For my yoke is easy and my burden is light."
*Here Jesus is talking about casting our burdens on him.


*Choose one of the following two verses to recite in your class. They are very similar.
Matthew 6:33 (NCV)
"Seek first God's kingdom and what God wants. Then all your other needs will be met as well."


Luke 12:30b–31
"but your Father already knows your needs. Seek the Kingdom of God above all else, and he will give you everything you need."


Luke 10:41–42 (NCV)
But the Lord answered her, "Martha, Martha, you are worried and upset about many things. Only one thing is important. Mary has chosen the better thing,"


Romans 15:13a (GW)
May God, the source of hope, fill you with joy and peace through your faith in him.


Proverbs 3:6 (LB)
In everything you do, put God first, and he will direct you and crown your efforts with success.


*Now as you move your yoga class into their relaxation posture tell them: Spend some time with the Lord and cast all your burdens on him because he cares for you. I will wake you when it is time.

\*Author's notes

The author has published a deck of Scripture Yoga Cards: "How to Receive God's Peace." You can find the cards at: http://christianyoga.com/yoga-books-decks.

## Chapter 13

# THE GREAT 'I AM'

It would be beneficial to read the Bible stories that correspond to some of these verses before your class. You can add information before or after the Scripture to enhance its meaning and extend the length of the class.

*I usually include this Scripture in the prayer before I begin the class.
Matthew 18:20 (GW)
"Where two or three have come together in my name, I am there among them."

*This is the first time in the New Testament God uses the name 'I Am.'
Before class read Exodus 3 about Moses and the burning bush.
Exodus 3:14 (RSV)
God said to Moses, "I AM WHO I AM." And he said, "Say this to the people of Israel, 'I AM has sent me to you.'"

John 6:35 (RSV)
Jesus said to them, "I am the bread of life; he who comes to me shall not hunger, and he who believes in me shall never thirst."

John 8:12 (RSV)
Again Jesus spoke to them, saying, "I am the light of the world; he who follows me will not walk in darkness, but will have the light of life."

John 15:5
"Yes, I am the vine; you are the branches. Those who remain in me, and I in them, will produce much fruit. For apart from me you can do nothing."

John 10:9 (NIV)
"I am the gate; whoever enters through me will be saved. They will come in and go out, and find pasture."

John 10:11 (NIV)
"I am the good shepherd. The good shepherd lays down his life for the sheep."

*After reciting these two verses, John 10:9, 11, I recite John 10:9-11 which includes the thief's purpose.
John 10:9–11
"Yes, I am the gate. Those who come in through me will be saved. They will come and go freely and will find good pastures. The thief's purpose is to steal and kill and destroy. My purpose is to give them a rich and satisfying life. I am the good shepherd. The good shepherd sacrifices his life for the sheep."

John 11:25 (NIV)
Jesus said to her, "I am the resurrection and the life. The one who believes in me will live, even though they die;"

*This is the same verse but from the Living Bible, which is a paraphrase of the Bible.
John 11:25-26 (LB)
Jesus told her, "I am the one who raises the dead and gives them life again. Anyone who believes in me, even though he dies like anyone else, shall live again. He is given eternal life for believing in me and shall never perish."

*Before the class, read John 14 and see the speculation from the disciple, Thomas.

John 14:6 (NIV)

Jesus answered, "I am the way and the truth and the life. No one comes to the Father except through me."

*During a yoga posture I recite all the different 'I am' statements I have spoken so far.

I am who I am.

I am the bread.

I am the light.

I am the vine.

I am the gate.

I am the good shepherd.

I am the resurrection and the life.

I am the way and the truth and the life.

*Before class, read John 18. The setting for this verse is in the Garden of Gethsemane.

John 18:4–6

Jesus fully realized all that was going to happen to him, so he stepped forward to meet them. "Who are you looking for?" he asked. "Jesus the Nazarene," they replied. "I Am he," Jesus said. (Judas, who betrayed him, was standing with them.) As Jesus said "I Am he," they all drew back and fell to the ground!

*Beforehand, read Mark 14:53-65 where the High Priest, Caiaphas, questions Jesus.

Mark 14:61–62

But Jesus was silent and made no reply. Then the high priest asked him, "Are you the Messiah, the Son of the Blessed One?" Jesus said, "I Am. And you will see the Son of Man seated in the place of power at God's right hand and coming on the clouds of heaven."

*I find it surprising that Jesus told them this.

Revelation 22:13
"I am the Alpha and the Omega, the First and the Last, the Beginning and the End."

Revelation 22:16b (NIV)
"I am the Root and the Offspring of David, and the bright Morning Star"

*Before class read John 4 about the Samaritan woman at the well.
John 4:26
Then Jesus told her, "I Am the Messiah!"

*Recite the last few 'I Am' statements.
I am the Alpha and the Omega.
I am the Root and Offspring of David.
I am the Messiah.

Matthew 28:20b (LB)
"And be sure of this, - that I am with you always, even to the end of the world."

*Author's notes

*Chapter 14*

# THE TABERNACLE

This theme demonstrates, through Scripture, how Jesus Christ fulfills all the parts of the Tabernacle or Temple (i.e., gate, light, bread, etc.). This theme was inspired by the Beth Moore study titled *A Woman's Heart: God's Dwelling Place* (1995).

*I read this first Scripture before beginning the class since it is long.
Hebrews 9:1–5a *Old Rules about Worship*
That first covenant between God and Israel had regulations for worship and a place of worship here on earth. There were two rooms in that Tabernacle. In the first room were a lampstand, a table, and sacred loaves of bread on the table. This room was called the Holy Place. Then there was a curtain, and behind the curtain was the second room called the Most Holy Place. In that room were a gold incense altar and a wooden chest called the Ark of the Covenant, which was covered with gold on all sides. Inside the Ark were a gold jar containing manna, Aaron's staff that sprouted leaves, and the stone tablets of the covenant. Above the Ark were the cherubim of divine glory, whose wings stretched out over the Ark's cover, the place of atonement.

*With the following verse I explain how God appeared as he gave the Ten Commandments.
Exodus 24:17 (GW)
To the Israelites, the glory of the LORD looked like a raging fire on top of the mountain.

*God said to Moses:
Exodus 25:8
"Have the people of Israel build me a holy sanctuary so I can live among them."

*God loved us so much that he, once again, wanted to live among us, similar to when he met with Adam.
Exodus 29:42b
at the Tabernacle entrance; there I will meet with you and speak with you.

Deuteronomy 1:33
who goes before you looking for the best places to camp, guiding you with a pillar of fire by night and a pillar of cloud by day.

Hebrews 9:23a
That is why the Tabernacle and everything in it, which were copies of things in heaven,
*Does the author mean this literally? Yes, he does.

*The next verse is John telling us about heaven:
Revelation 11:19a
Then, in heaven, the Temple of God was opened and the Ark of his covenant could be seen inside the Temple.

*You must pass through a gate before you entered into the courtyard of the Temple.
John 10:9a (NIV)
"I am the gate; whoever enters through me will be saved."
Jesus is the gate.

*Once inside the Temple courtyard there was a large altar.
Hebrews 10:11–12a
Under the old covenant, the priest stands and ministers before the altar day after day, offering the same sacrifices again and again, which can never take away sins. But our High Priest offered himself to God as a single sacrifice for sins, good for all time.

Hebrews 10:10
For God's will was for us to be made holy by the sacrifice of the body of Jesus Christ, once for all time.

*In the Temple courtyard, between the altar and the Temple entrance, there was a wash basin, called a Laver. Jesus must wash us clean through his sacrifice, as he explained to Peter.
John 13:8
"No," Peter protested, "you will never ever wash my feet!" Jesus replied, "Unless I wash you, you won't belong to me."

*Inside the Temple, a single lampstand lit the first room in the Temple. This room was called the Holy Place.
John 8:12 *Jesus, the Light of the World*
Jesus spoke to the people once more and said, "I am the light of the world. If you follow me, you won't have to walk in darkness, because you will have the light that leads to life."

*Inside the Holy Place was a table with 12 loaves of the Bread of the Presence, which represented the 12 tribes of Israel.
John 6:35a (NCV)
Then Jesus said, "I am the bread that gives life. Whoever comes to me will never be hungry"

*The most holy curtain separated the Holy Place from the second room called the Most Holy Place.

Hebrews 10:19–22 (NCV) *Continue to Trust God*

So, brothers and sisters, we are completely free to enter the Most Holy Place without fear because of the blood of Jesus' death. We can enter through a new and living way that Jesus opened for us. It leads through the curtain—Christ's body. And since we have a great priest over God's house, let us come near to God with a sincere heart and a sure faith, because we have been made free from a guilty conscience, and our bodies have been washed with pure water.

*The following is the same verse as above, but in the New Living Translation.

Hebrews 10:19–22   *A Call to Persevere*

And so, dear brothers and sisters, we can boldly enter heaven's Most Holy Place because of the blood of Jesus. By his death, Jesus opened a new and life-giving way through the curtain into the Most Holy Place. And since we have a great High Priest who rules over God's house, let us go right into the presence of God with sincere hearts fully trusting him. For our guilty consciences have been sprinkled with Christ's blood to make us clean, and our bodies have been washed with pure water.

*Through Jesus' sacrifice and the shedding of his innocent blood we have atonement. From a Christian perspective, atonement is the reconciliation between God and people brought about by the death of Jesus Christ.

Leviticus 16:15a–16a

"Then Aaron must slaughter the first goat as a sin offering for the people and carry its blood behind the inner curtain. There he will sprinkle the goat's blood over the atonement cover and in front of it. Through this process, he will purify the Most Holy Place"

*Inside the Most Holy Place there was an Altar of Incense.

This is John telling us what is going on in heaven.

Revelation 8:3–4a

Then another angel with a gold incense burner came and stood at the altar. And a great amount of incense was given to him to mix with the prayers of God's people as an offering on the gold altar before the throne. The smoke of the incense, mixed with the prayers of God's holy people, ascended up to God from the altar.

*Christ is interceding for us.

Romans 8:34

Who then will condemn us? No one—for Christ Jesus died for us and was raised to life for us, and he is sitting in the place of honor at God's right hand, pleading for us.

Psalm 141:2

Accept my prayer as incense offered to you, and my upraised hands as an evening offering.

*The Ark of the Covenant:

Inside: stone tablets, a jar of manna, and Aaron's rod that budded almonds.

Cover: pure gold with Cherubim wings covering it.

Atonement Cover: where God told Moses he would meet with him and talk to him, between the Cherubim.

Exodus 25:22a

I will meet with you there and talk to you from above the atonement cover between the gold cherubim that hover over the Ark of the Covenant.

Psalm 99:1

The LORD is king! Let the nations tremble! He sits on his throne between the cherubim. Let the whole earth quake!

*The Ark of the Covenant was shaped like a coffin. In this verse, we see where the angels were at the foot and head where Jesus' dead body had laid.

John 20:11–12 *Jesus Appears to Mary Magdalene*
Mary was standing outside the tomb crying, and as she wept, she stooped and looked in. She saw two white-robed angels, one sitting at the head and the other at the foot of the place where the body of Jesus had been lying.

*The Tabernacle was God's home on earth. He filled it with his glory. Almost 500 years later, King Solomon built the Temple, which replaced the Tabernacle.
Nearly 500 years later, Jesus taught at the second Temple.
After Jesus was crucified and rose from the dead God no longer needed a physical building, because now God's Temple is the body of his believers, his church! And he dwells in us through his Holy Spirit!

Revelation 1:6a
He has made us a Kingdom of priests for God his Father.
*This is a great privilege, as well as, responsibility.

2 Corinthians 2:14b - 15a (NIV) *Ministers of the New Covenant*
Now he uses us to spread the knowledge of Christ everywhere, like a sweet perfume. For we are to God the pleasing aroma of Christ.

2 Corinthians 2:15–16a
Our lives are a Christ-like fragrance rising up to God. But this fragrance is perceived differently by those who are being saved and by those who are perishing. To those who are perishing, we are a dreadful smell of death and doom. But to those who are being saved, we are a life-giving perfume.

*Author's notes

## *Chapter 15*

# WORSHIP AND GLORY

Revelation 4:11a
"You are worthy, O Lord our God, to receive glory and honor and power. For you created all things,"

Psalm 150:6
Let everything that breathes sing praises to the LORD! Praise the LORD!

Psalm 113:3 (LB)
Praise him from sunrise to sunset!

Psalm 42:1
As the deer longs for streams of water, so I long for you, O God.

Galatians 4:6
And because we are his children, God has sent the Spirit of his Son into our hearts, prompting us to call out, "Abba, Father."

John 4:24
"For God is Spirit, so those who worship him must worship in spirit and in truth."

1 Corinthians 2:16b (NCV)
But we have the mind of Christ.

*Read chapter 2 of Daniel and explain in your words why Daniel praised God through this prayer:

Daniel 2:20–23

He said, "Praise the name of God forever and ever, for he has all wisdom and power. He controls the course of world events; he removes kings and sets up other kings. He gives wisdom to the wise and knowledge to the scholars. He reveals deep and mysterious things and knows what lies hidden in darkness, though he is surrounded by light. I thank and praise you, God of my ancestors, for you have given me wisdom and strength. You have told me what we asked of you and revealed to us what the king demanded."

2 Corinthians 4:17

For our present troubles are small and won't last very long. Yet they produce for us a glory that vastly outweighs them and will last forever!

James 1:2–3  *Faith and Endurance*

Dear brothers and sisters, when troubles come your way, consider it an opportunity for great joy. For you know that when your faith is tested, your endurance has a chance to grow.

Romans 8:18 *The Future Glory*

Yet what we suffer now is nothing compared to the glory he will reveal to us later.

Isaiah 43:7

"Bring all who claim me as their God, for I have made them for my glory. It was I who created them."

2 Corinthians 1:3b–4 *God Offers Comfort to All*

God is our merciful Father and the source of all comfort. He comforts us in all our troubles so that we can comfort others. When they are troubled, we will be able to give them the same comfort God has given us.

*Author's notes

# Chapter 16

# ATONEMENT AND RIGHTEOUSNESS

Isaiah 1:18b
says the LORD. "Though your sins are like scarlet, I will make them as white as snow. Though they are red like crimson, I will make them as white as wool."

*The 'righteous servant' in the following verse is the Messiah, Jesus Christ.
Isaiah 53:11b
And because of his experience, my righteous servant will make it possible for many to be counted righteous, for he will bear all their sins.
*Chapter 53 of Isaiah speaks of the Messiah. A Jewish man informed me that, for them, the book of Isaiah did not include this chapter. He felt mislead because this chapter points directly to Jesus.

2 Corinthians 5:21 (LB)
For God took the sinless Christ and poured into him our sins. Then, in exchange, he poured God's goodness into us!
*See explanation of this verse in Chapter 7: The Greatest Gift of them All–Love.

John 13:8 (NCV)

Peter said, "No, you will never wash my feet." Jesus answered, "If I don't wash your feet, you are not one of my people."

*Jesus must wash us clean through his sacrifice.

Hebrews 8:12 (NCV)

I will forgive them for the wicked things they did, and I will not remember their sins

anymore" (a New Testament quote from Jeremiah 31:31–34).

Ephesians 1:11a (LB)

Moreover, because of what Christ has done we have become gifts to God that he delights in,

*Remember, God delights in you!

Psalm 18:19b (NIV)

he rescued me because he delighted in me.

*This is one of my favorite verses. It is a key to happiness while on this earth.

2 Corinthians 5:15 (NIV)

And he died for all, that those who live should no longer live for themselves but for him who died for them and was raised again.

1 John 4:9–10 (NCV)

This is how God showed his love to us: He sent his one and only Son into the world so that we could have life through him. This is what real love is: It is not our love for God; it is God's love for us. He sent his Son to die in our place to take away our sins.

John 16:33b
"Here on earth you will have many trials and sorrows. But take heart, because I have overcome the world."
*Jesus defeated sin, death and, ultimately, Satan.

Matthew 18:14b (NIV)
"your Father in heaven is not willing that any of these little ones should perish."

John 3:16 (NIV)
For God so loved the world that he gave his one and only Son, that whoever believes in him shall not perish but have eternal life.

2 Peter 3:9 (LB)
He isn't really being slow about his promised return, even though it sometimes seems that way. But he is waiting, for the good reason that he is not willing that any should perish, and he is giving more time for sinners to repent.

Matthew 12:30a (NIV)
"Whoever is not with me is against me,"

1 John 2:2a (LB)
He is the one who took God's wrath against our sins upon himself, and brought us into fellowship with God; and he is the forgiveness for our sins
*Jesus is the forgiveness of our sins.

Psalm 103:1-5 (LB)
I bless the holy name of God with all my heart. Yes, I will bless the Lord and not forget the glorious things he does for me. He forgives all

my sins. He heals me. He ransoms me from hell. He surrounds me with lovingkindness and tender mercies. He fills my life with good things!

Hebrews 10:10 (GW)
We have been set apart as holy because Jesus Christ did what God wanted him to do by sacrificing his body once and for all.
*One sacrifice, for all, for all times.


*Author's notes

# Chapter 17

# PRAYING AND BELIEVING

I have produced the Christian yoga DVD, *What the Bible Says About Prayer*, using this theme.

Mark 1:35
Before daybreak the next morning, Jesus got up and went out to an isolated place to pray.

Psalm 66:18
If I had not confessed the sin in my heart, the Lord would not have listened.

Psalm 139:23–24a
Search me, O God, and know my heart; test me and know my anxious thoughts. Point out anything in me that offends you,

*This is a very long Scripture I recently added to this theme. Therefore, I would use it only after you are familiar with this lesson. It is a powerful prayer of repentance by King David.
Psalm 51:1–17 *For the choir director: A psalm of David, regarding the time Nathan the prophet came to him after David had committed adultery with Bathsheba and killed Uriah.*
Have mercy on me, O God, because of your unfailing love. Because of your great compassion, blot out the stain of my sins. Wash me clean from my guilt. Purify me from my sin. For I recognize my rebellion; it haunts

me day and night. Against you, and you alone, have I sinned; I have done what is evil in your sight. You will be proved right in what you say, and your judgment against me is just. For I was born a sinner— yes, from the moment my mother conceived me. But you desire honesty from the womb, teaching me wisdom even there. Purify me from my sins, and I will be clean; wash me, and I will be whiter than snow. Oh, give me back my joy again; you have broken me— now let me rejoice. Don't keep looking at my sins. Remove the stain of my guilt. Create in me a clean heart, O God. Renew a loyal spirit within me. Do not banish me from your presence, and don't take your Holy Spirit from me. Restore to me the joy of your salvation, and make me willing to obey you. Then I will teach your ways to rebels, and they will return to you. Forgive me for shedding blood, O God who saves; then I will joyfully sing of your forgiveness. Unseal my lips, O Lord, that my mouth may praise you. You do not desire a sacrifice, or I would offer one. You do not want a burnt offering. The sacrifice you desire is a broken spirit. You will not reject a broken and repentant heart, O God.

Isaiah 59:1–2 *Warnings against Sin*
Listen! The LORD's arm is not too weak to save you, nor is his ear too deaf to hear you call. It's your sins that have cut you off from God. Because of your sins, he has turned away and will not listen anymore. *It is apparent from this verse that God will not listen to you if you are sinful. A person needs to repent.

1 John 3:21–22
Dear friends, if we don't feel guilty, we can come to God with bold confidence. And we will receive from him whatever we ask because we obey him and do the things that please him.

John 15:7 (LB)
"But if you stay in me and obey my commands, you may ask any request you like, and it will be granted!"

*Staying with me or abiding in Christ is the awareness that God is always present and listening to you. Invite Jesus to be your companion. Recognize that he is present and live in his presence.

*God has promised that when we walk faithfully with him and when he becomes an integral part of our everyday lives, his spirit will guide us in such a way that his protection will surround everything we say and do.

*God wants to take us gently by the hand and lead us so that we are blessed and he is glorified.

John 4:24
"For God is Spirit, so those who worship him must worship in spirit and in truth."

Matthew 21:22
"You can pray for anything, and if you have faith, you will receive it."

*This is a story about faith:
Matthew 8:5–8, 10, 13 *The Faith of a Roman Officer*
When Jesus returned to Capernaum, a Roman officer came and pleaded with him, "Lord, my young servant lies in bed, paralyzed and in terrible pain." Jesus said, "I will come and heal him."
But the officer said, "Lord, I am not worthy to have you come into my home. Just say the word from where you are, and my servant will be healed."
When Jesus heard this, he was amazed. Turning to those who were following him, he said, "I tell you the truth, I haven't seen faith like this in all Israel!"
Then Jesus said to the Roman officer, "Go back home. Because you believed, it has happened." And the young servant was healed that same hour.

Mark 11:24

"I tell you, you can pray for anything, and if you believe that you've received it, it will be yours."

*But do your prayers focus on God's kingdom and God's will?

Hebrews 11:1  *Great Examples of Faith*

Faith is the confidence that what we hope for will actually happen; it gives us assurance about things we cannot see.

John 16:23–24

"At that time you won't need to ask me for anything. I tell you the truth, you will ask the Father directly, and he will grant your request because you use my name. You haven't done this before. Ask, using my name, and you will receive, and you will have abundant joy."

*After Jesus' resurrection, any believer can approach God directly because Jesus has made us acceptable to God. So use the name of Jesus when you pray.

*This setting of this verse was the Garden of Gethsemane.

Matthew 26:39

He went on a little farther and bowed with his face to the ground, praying, "My Father! If it is possible, let this cup of suffering be taken away from me. Yet I want your will to be done, not mine."

*Prayer is the link between the Father's will and our work on earth. That is why Jesus got up early and spent time with his Father. We should too.

*Many of these verses contain an "If ... then" statement:

1. If we confessed the sins in our hearts
2. Because we obey him
3. Because we do the things that please Him
4. If you abide in Christ
5. If you have faith in what you pray about

6. If you ask in the name of Jesus

7. Asking for God's will, not your own

*When Peter was about to be tempted by Satan, what did Jesus do?

Luke 22:31–32 *Jesus Predicts Peter's Denial*

"Simon, Simon, Satan has asked to sift each of you like wheat. But I have pleaded in prayer for you, Simon, that your faith should not fail. So when you have repented and turned to me again, strengthen your brothers."

*I believe prayer is more important than we realize, it enters the unseen spiritual realm. We should pray more.

Matthew 18:19-20 (NASB95)

"I also tell you this: If two of you agree here on earth concerning anything you ask, my Father in heaven will do it for you. For where two or three have gathered together in My name, I am there in their midst."

Romans 8:26–27

And the Holy Spirit helps us in our weakness. For example, we don't know what God wants us to pray for. But the Holy Spirit prays for us with groanings that cannot be expressed in words. And the Father who knows all hearts knows what the Spirit is saying, for the Spirit pleads for us believers in harmony with God's own will.

*If I am praying for a situation I do not know a lot about, I ask the Holy Spirit to pray in harmony with God's will.

Hebrews 4:16

So let us come boldly to the throne of our gracious God. There we will receive his mercy, and we will find grace to help us when we need it most.

James 5:13  *The Power of Prayer*
Are any of you suffering hardships? You should pray. Are any of you happy? You should sing praises.

James 5:16b
The earnest prayer of a righteous person has great power and produces wonderful results.

John 20:29
Then Jesus told him, "You believe because you have seen me. Blessed are those who believe without seeing me."

Luke 18:8b (LB)
"When I, the Messiah, return, how many will I find who have faith [and are praying]?"

*The corresponding DVD, *What the Bible Says About Prayer*, can be found on ChristianYoga.com.


*Author's notes

# Chapter 18

# HOW TO BE GOD'S LIGHT AND BEAR HIS FRUIT

Matthew 5:16 (GW)
"In the same way let your light shine in front of people. Then they will see the good that you do and praise your Father in heaven."

Philippians 2:15–16
so that no one can criticize you. Live clean, innocent lives as children of God, shining like bright lights in a world full of crooked and perverse people. Hold firmly to the word of life; then, on the day of Christ's return, I will be proud that I did not run the race in vain and that my work was not useless.

Matthew 5:14 (LB)
"You are the world's light — a city on a hill, glowing in the night for all to see."

Psalm 104:1–2a (GW)
Praise the LORD, my soul! O LORD my God, you are very great. You are clothed with splendor and majesty. You cover yourself with light as though it were a robe.

1 John 1:5b *Living in the Light*
God is light, and there is no darkness in him at all.

Ephesians 5:8–9
For once you were full of darkness, but now you have light from the Lord. So live as people of light! For this light within you produces only what is good and right and true.

2 Corinthians 4:7
We now have this light shining in our hearts, but we ourselves are like fragile clay jars containing this great treasure. This makes it clear that our great power is from God, not from ourselves.

Romans 8:10
And Christ lives within you, so even though your body will die because of sin, the Spirit gives you life because you have been made right with God.

Romans 8:11
The Spirit of God, who raised Jesus from the dead, lives in you. And just as God raised Christ Jesus from the dead, he will give life to your mortal bodies by this same Spirit living within you.

2 Samuel 22:29 (GW)
O Lord, you are my lamp. The Lord turns my darkness into light.

John 15:16a
"You didn't choose me. I chose you. I appointed you to go and produce lasting fruit,"
*Many times God will lead me to repeat this verse several times throughout the class.

Isaiah 55:10–11
"The rain and snow come down from the heavens and stay on the ground to water the earth. They cause the grain to grow, producing seed for the farmer and bread for the hungry. It is the same with my word. I send it

out, and it always produces fruit. It will accomplish all I want it to, and it will prosper everywhere I send it."

1 Corinthians 3:6–7
Paul says, I planted the seed in your hearts, and Apollos watered it, but it was God who made it grow. It's not important who does the planting, or who does the watering. What's important is that God makes the seed grow. For we are both God's workers. And you are God's field. You are God's building.
*It is amazing to think we can be God's workers!

Galatians 5:22
But the Holy Spirit produces this kind of fruit in our lives: love, joy, peace, patience, kindness, goodness, faithfulness,

John 20:21b
"As the Father has sent me, so I am sending you."

Matthew 28:19
"Therefore, go and make disciples of all the nations, baptizing them in the name of the Father and the Son and the Holy Spirit."

John 15:1  *Jesus, the True Vine*
"I am the true grapevine, and my Father is the gardener. Yes, I am the vine; you are the branches. Those who remain in me, and I in them, will produce much fruit. For apart from me you can do nothing"


*Author's notes

# Chapter 19

# DECISIONS, OBEDIENCE, AND JOY

Proverbs 2:9 (LB)
He shows how to distinguish right from wrong, how to find the right decision every time.

John 10:27 (NIV)
"My sheep listen to my voice; I know them, and they follow me."

James 1:5 (GW)
If any of you needs wisdom to know what you should do, you should ask God, and he will give it to you. God is generous to everyone and doesn't find fault with them.

Psalm 37:23
The LORD directs the steps of the godly. He delights in every detail of their lives.

Proverbs 3:6
Seek his will in all you do, and he will show you which path to take.

Psalm 37:4 (NIV)
Take delight in the LORD, and he will give you the desires of your heart.

Romans 12:2 (NIV)

Do not conform to the pattern of this world, but be transformed by the renewing of your mind. Then you will be able to test and approve what God's will is—his good, pleasing and perfect will.

Romans 12:2 (NCV)

Do not be shaped by this world; instead be changed within by a new way of thinking. Then you will be able to decide what God wants for you; you will know what is good and pleasing to him and what is perfect.

Philippians 4:13

For I can do everything through Christ, who gives me strength.

John 8:31-32 (LB)

Jesus said them, "You are truly my disciples if you live as I tell you to, and you will know the truth, and the truth will set you free."

1 John 5:3–4

Loving God means keeping his commandments, and his commandments are not burdensome. For every child of God defeats this evil world, and we achieve this victory through our faith.

1 John 5:3–4 (LB)

Loving God means doing what he tells you to do, and really, that isn't hard at all; for every child of God can obey him, defeating sin and evil pleasure by trusting Christ to help him

Philippians 2:13

For God is working in you, giving you the desire and the power to do what pleases him.

John 15:10–11

"When you obey my commandments, you remain in my love, just as I obey my Father's commandments and remain in his love. I have told you these things so that you will be filled with my joy. Yes, your joy will overflow!"

*Compare and contrast Jonah, who did not obey God, and Paul, who did obey.

Philippians 4:11b (NIV)

for I have learned to be content whatever the circumstances.

Philippians 4:11b (ESV)

for I have learned in whatever situation I am to be content.

2 Chronicles 16:9a (NCV)

The LORD searches all the earth for people who have given themselves completely to him. He wants to make them strong.

*Author's notes

# Chapter 20

# SERVING AND TITHING

Proverbs 3:6 (LB)
In everything you do, put God first, and he will direct you and crown your efforts with success.

*So, how do you remember to put God first? The next verse tells you how.
Deuteronomy 14:23b (LB)
The purpose of tithing is to teach you always to put God first in your lives.

2 Corinthians 9:7b
You must each decide in your heart how much to give. And don't give reluctantly or in response to pressure. "For God loves a person who gives cheerfully."

Malachi 3:10
Bring all the tithes into the storehouse so there will be enough food in my Temple. If you do," says the LORD of Heaven's Armies, "I will open the windows of heaven for you. I will pour out a blessing so great you won't have enough room to take it in! Try it! Put me to the test!
*There are many different types of blessings.

Proverbs 19:17 (NIV)
Whoever is kind to the poor lends to the LORD, and he will reward them for what they have done.

Ephesians 6:7
Work with enthusiasm, as though you were working for the Lord rather than for people.

1 Peter 4:10a (NIV)
Each of you should use whatever gift you have received to serve others, *Are you serving God with your spiritual gift?

Romans 12:6-8
In his grace, God has given us different gifts for doing certain things well. So if God has given you the ability to prophesy, speak out with as much faith as God has given you. If your gift is serving others, serve them well. If you are a teacher, teach well. If your gift is to encourage others, be encouraging. If it is giving, give generously. If God has given you leadership ability, take the responsibility seriously. And if you have a gift for showing kindness to others, do it gladly.

1 Corinthians 12:7-10
A spiritual gift is given to each of us so we can help each other. To one person the Spirit gives the ability to give wise advice; to another the same Spirit gives a message of special knowledge. The same Spirit gives great faith to another, and to someone else the one Spirit gives the gift of healing. He gives one person the power to perform miracles, and another the ability to prophesy. He gives someone else the ability to discern whether a message is from the Spirit of God or from another spirit. Still another person is given the ability to speak in unknown languages, while another is given the ability to interpret what is being said.

3 John 1:8 (NIV)
We ought therefore to show hospitality to such people so that we may work together for the truth.

Joshua 24:15b (NIV)
"But as for me and my household, we will serve the LORD."

Galatians 6:9
So let's not get tired of doing what is good. At just the right time we will reap a harvest of blessing if we don't give up.

2 Chronicles 16:9a
The eyes of the LORD search the whole earth in order to strengthen those whose hearts are fully committed to him.

*Author's notes

# Chapter 21

# MARRIAGE AND CHILDREN

Genesis 2:18 (NIV)
The LORD God said, "It is not good for the man to be alone. I will make a helper suitable for him."
*Man alone was not complete. Therefore, God made him a helper, woman.
*Helper means "one who provides aid or relief, most notably the Lord" (Logos Bible Software, 2004). The same word (helper) is used several other times in the Bible to demonstrate how God is our Savior. Interesting!

Genesis 2:24 (NIV)
That is why a man leaves his father and mother and is united to his wife, and they become one flesh.
*The husband is to put his wife before his parents.

Ephesians 5:21 *Spirit-Guided Relationships: Wives and Husbands*
And further, submit to one another out of reverence for Christ.
*Both are to submit to each other!

Ephesians 5:22–24 (GW) *Paul's Advice to Wives and Husbands*
Wives, place yourselves under your husbands' authority as you have placed yourselves under the Lord's authority. The husband is the head of his wife as Christ is the head of the church. It is his body, and he is

its Savior. As the church is under Christ's authority, so wives are under their husbands' authority in everything.

*The wife can disagree with her husband but should yield to his leadership in the final decision on important matters.

Ephesians 5:25, 28, 29a (GW)

Husbands, love your wives as Christ loved the church and gave his life for it.

So husbands must love their wives as they love their own bodies. A man who loves his wife loves himself. No one ever hated his own body.

*I am not sure which is more difficult: being under your husband's authority or loving your wife as you love your own body and as Christ loved the church.

Ephesians 5:33

So again I say, each man must love his wife as he loves himself, and the wife must respect her husband.

*Treating your husband with respect helps God's love flow from your husband to you.

Ephesians 5:30–31 (GW)

We are parts of his body. That's why a man will leave his father and mother and be united with his wife, and the two will be one.

*A husband and wife become one flesh. They are better together than apart. When they fight each other they are fighting themselves.

Genesis 3:16

Then he said to the woman, "I will sharpen the pain of your pregnancy, and in pain you will give birth. And you will desire to control your husband, but he will rule over you."

*The curse heightens the conflict in marriages.

Colossians 3:19 (NIV)
Husbands, love your wives and do not be harsh with them.

1 Peter 3:1–2 *Wives*
In the same way, you wives must accept the authority of your husbands. Then, even if some refuse to obey the Good News, your godly lives will speak to them without any words. They will be won over by observing your pure and reverent lives.
*Don't preach to your husband. Instead, have him observe God working in your life. Work on your own life, not his and pray.

1 Peter 3:7 *Husbands*
In the same way, you husbands must give honor to your wives. Treat your wife with understanding as you live together. She may be weaker than you are, but she is your equal partner in God's gift of new life. Treat her as you should so your prayers will not be hindered.

Proverbs 14:1
A wise woman builds her home, but a foolish woman tears it down with her own hands.
*Be wise and pray for your husband and children. Ask God to intervene in their lives.

Proverbs 31:10
Who can find a virtuous and capable wife? She is more precious than rubies.

Proverbs 31: 11b
She will greatly enrich his (her husbands) life.

Proverbs 31:26
When she speaks, her words are wise, and she gives instruction with kindness.
*Do you give instruction with kindness?

Proverbs 31:27a
She carefully watches everything in her household

Proverbs 31:30b
but a woman who fears the Lord will be greatly praised.
*In this verse fear means worshipful submission, reverential awe, and obedient respect (Logos Bible software, 2004).

Matthew 19:14
But Jesus said, "Let the children come to me. Don't stop them! For the Kingdom of Heaven belongs to those who are like these children."
*I believe Jesus was talking about a child's steadfast faith.

Proverbs 22:6 (NCV)
Train children to live the right way, and when they are old, they will not stray from it.
*When you are in the trenches raising your little ones this does not seem possible but have faith because it is true!

Psalm 127:3
Children are a gift from the LORD; they are a reward from him.
*Did you know that your child is God's gift to you?

*Author's notes

# *Chapter 22*

# GOD'S MIGHTY ANGELS

I produced the Christian yoga DVD, *God's Mighty Angels*, using this theme.

*This is what the angels say as they surround the throne of God:
Revelation 4:8
"Holy, holy, holy is the Lord God, the Almighty— the one who always was, who is, and who is still to come."

Isaiah 6:3 (NIV)
And they were calling to one another: "Holy, holy, holy is the LORD Almighty;
the whole earth is full of his glory."

Nehemiah 9:6
the angels of heaven worship you.

*This verse is talking about salvation.
1 Peter 1:12 (LB)
And now at last this good news has been plainly announced to all of us. And it is all so strange and wonderful that even the angels in heaven would give a great deal to know more about it.

Hebrews 1:14 (NCV)
All the angels are spirits who serve God and are sent to help those who will receive salvation.

*The guardian angel saying comes from this verse.

Matthew 18:10

"Beware that you don't look down on any of these little ones. For I tell you that in heaven their angels are always in the presence of my heavenly Father."

Psalm 91:11–12

For he will order his angels to protect you wherever you go. They will hold you up with their hands so you won't even hurt your foot on a stone.

Matthew 26:53–54

"Don't you realize that I could ask my Father for thousands of angels to protect us, and he would send them instantly? But if I did, how would the Scriptures be fulfilled that describe what must happen now?"

*Now we will look at stories from the Old and New Testament regarding angels.

Daniel 6:19–23

Very early the next morning, the king got up and hurried out to the lions' den. When he got there, he called out in anguish, "Daniel, servant of the living God! Was your God, whom you serve so faithfully, able to rescue you from the lions?"

Daniel answered, "Long live the king! My God sent his angel to shut the lions' mouths so that they would not hurt me, for I have been found innocent in his sight. And I have not wronged you, Your Majesty."

The king was overjoyed and ordered that Daniel be lifted from the den. Not a scratch was found on him, for he had trusted in his God.

Acts 12:5–10 *Peter's Miraculous Escape from Prison*

But while Peter was in prison, the church prayed very earnestly for him. The night before Peter was to be placed on trial, he was asleep, fastened with two chains between two soldiers. Others stood guard at the prison gate. Suddenly, there was a bright light in the cell, and an angel of the Lord stood before Peter. The angel struck him on the side to awaken him and said, "Quick! Get up!" And the chains fell off his wrists. Then the angel told him, "Get dressed and put on your sandals." And he did. "Now put on your coat and follow me," the angel ordered.

So Peter left the cell, following the angel. But all the time he thought it was a vision. He didn't realize it was actually happening. They passed the first and second guard posts and came to the iron gate leading to the city, and this opened for them all by itself. So they passed through and started walking down the street, and then the angel suddenly left him.

Hebrews 1:7 (LB)
God speaks of his angels as messengers swift as the wind and as servants made of flaming fire.

Luke 1:11–13
While Zechariah was in the sanctuary, an angel of the Lord appeared to him, standing to the right of the incense altar. Zechariah was shaken and overwhelmed with fear when he saw him. But the angel said, "Don't be afraid, Zechariah! God has heard your prayer. Your wife, Elizabeth, will give you a son, and you are to name him John."

Psalm 89:8 (LB)
O Jehovah, Commander of the heavenly armies

Psalm 103:20
Praise the LORD, you angels, you mighty ones who carry out his plans, listening for each of his commands.

Revelation 22:8–9
I, John, am the one who heard and saw all these things. And when I heard and saw them, I fell down to worship at the feet of the angel who showed them to me. But he said, "No, don't worship me. I am a servant

of God, just like you and your brothers the prophets, as well as all who obey what is written in this book. Worship only God!"

Matthew 28:2–3
Suddenly there was a great earthquake! For an angel of the Lord came down from heaven, rolled aside the stone, and sat on it. His face shone like lightning, and his clothing was as white as snow.

Luke 15:10 (NIV)
"In the same way, I tell you, there is rejoicing in the presence of the angels of God over one sinner who repents."

Revelation 5:11 (NIV)
Then I looked and heard the voice of many angels, numbering thousands upon thousands, and ten thousand times ten thousand. They encircled the throne

Luke 2:8–11, 13-14  *The Shepherds and Angels*
That night there were shepherds staying in the fields nearby, guarding their flocks of sheep. Suddenly, an angel of the Lord appeared among them, and the radiance of the Lord's glory surrounded them. They were terrified, but the angel reassured them. "Don't be afraid!" he said. "I bring you good news that will bring great joy to all people. The Savior—yes, the Messiah, the Lord—has been born today in Bethlehem, the city of David!"
Suddenly, the angel was joined by a vast host of others—the armies of heaven—praising God and saying, "Glory to God in highest heaven, and peace on earth to those with whom God is pleased."

Matthew 24:31
"And he will send out his angels with the mighty blast of a trumpet, and they will gather his chosen ones from all over the world—from the farthest ends of the earth and heaven."

Matthew 16:27

"For the Son of Man will come with his angels in the glory of his Father and will judge all people according to their deeds."

Matthew 13:41–43

"The Son of Man will send his angels, and they will remove from his Kingdom everything that causes sin and all who do evil. And the angels will throw them into the fiery furnace, where there will be weeping and gnashing of teeth. Then the righteous will shine like the sun in their Father's Kingdom. Anyone with ears to hear should listen and understand!"

*Author's notes

*You can purchase the *God's Mighty Angel* DVD at http://christianyoga. com

# Chapter 23

# ANGELIC VISITATIONS SURROUNDING THE BIRTH OF CHRIST

I use this theme in December as it prepares our hearts and minds for the celebration of Christmas and its true meaning.

Luke 1:5, 7
When Herod was king of Judea, there was a Jewish priest named Zechariah. He was a member of the priestly order of Abijah, and his wife, Elizabeth, was also. They had no children because Elizabeth was unable to conceive, and they were both very old.

Luke 1:8-10
One day Zechariah was serving God in the Temple, for his order was on duty that week.
As was the custom of the priests, he was chosen by lot to enter the sanctuary of the Lord and burn incense. While the incense was being burned, a great crowd stood outside, praying.

*Once in a lifetime a priest was chosen to offer incense at the Temple in Jerusalem. This was Zachariah's turn.
Luke 1:11–13 (The Message)
Unannounced, an angel of God appeared just to the right of the altar of incense. Zachariah was paralyzed in fear. But the angel reassured him,

"Don't fear, Zachariah. Your prayer has been heard. Elizabeth, your wife, will bear a son by you. You are to name him John."

Luke 1:18-20a
Zechariah said to the angel, "How can I be sure this will happen? I'm an old man now, and my wife is also well along in years." Then the angel said, "I am Gabriel! I stand in the very presence of God. It was he who sent me to bring you this good news! But now, since you didn't believe what I said, you will be silent and unable to speak until the child is born.
*Two thoughts are fascinating:
1. Zechariah lacked faith.
2. Gabriel had the power and authority to make Zechariah mute because of his faithlessness.

Luke 1:21-22
Meanwhile, the people were waiting for Zechariah to come out of the sanctuary, wondering why he was taking so long. When he finally did come out, he couldn't speak to them. Then they realized from his gestures and his silence that he must have seen a vision in the sanctuary.

*Six to seven months later Gabriel visits Mary, which is the second angelic visitation.
Luke 1:26–31 *The Birth of Jesus Foretold*
In the sixth month of Elizabeth's pregnancy, God sent the angel Gabriel to Nazareth, a village in Galilee, to a virgin named Mary. She was engaged to be married to a man named Joseph, a descendant of King David. Gabriel appeared to her and said, "Greetings, favored woman! The Lord is with you!"
Confused and disturbed, Mary tried to think what the angel could mean. "Don't be afraid, Mary," the angel told her, "for you have found favor with God! You will conceive and give birth to a son, and you will name him Jesus."

Luke 1:34-35

Mary asked the angel, "But how can this happen? I am a virgin." The angel replied, "The Holy Spirit will come upon you, and the power of the Most High will overshadow you. So the baby to be born will be holy, and he will be called the Son of God.

*Mary did not question Gabriel because she lacked faith but from a lack of understanding.

Luke 1:36-37

What's more, your relative Elizabeth has become pregnant in her old age! People used to say she was barren, but she has conceived a son and is now in her sixth month. For nothing is impossible with God.

Luke 1: 38

Mary responded, "I am the Lord's servant. May everything you have said about me come true." And then the angel left her.

Luke 1:39

A few days later Mary hurried to the hill country of Judea, to the town

Luke 1:56

Mary stayed with Elizabeth about three months and then went back to her own home.

*I explain how Joseph was going to break off their engagement quietly when:
Matthew 1:20

As he considered this, an angel of the Lord appeared to him in a dream. "Joseph, son of David," the angel said, "do not be afraid to take Mary as your wife. For the child within her was conceived by the Holy Spirit."
*This was the third angelic visitation.

## Luke 2:1, 3-4

At that time the Roman emperor, Augustus, decreed that a census should be taken throughout the Roman Empire. All returned to their own ancestral towns to register for this census. And because Joseph was a descendant of King David, he had to go to Bethlehem in Judea, David's ancient home. He traveled there from the village of Nazareth in Galilee.

## Luke 2:5-6

He took with him Mary, his fiancée, who was now obviously pregnant. And while they were there, the time came for her baby to be born.

## Luke 2:8–14 (NKJV) *The Angels Announce Jesus to the Shepherds*

Now there were in the same country shepherds living out in the fields, keeping watch over their flock by night. And behold, an angel of the Lord stood before them, and the glory of the Lord shone around them, and they were greatly afraid. Then the angel said to them, "Do not be afraid, for behold, I bring you good tidings of great joy which will be to all people. For there is born to you this day in the city of David a Savior, who is Christ the Lord. And this *will be* the sign to you: You will find a Babe wrapped in swaddling cloths, lying in a manger."

And suddenly there was with the angel a multitude of the heavenly host praising God and saying: "Glory to God in the highest, And on earth peace, goodwill toward men!"

*This was the fourth angelic visit.

## Matthew 2:1–5 *Visitors from the East*

Jesus was born in Bethlehem in Judea, during the reign of King Herod. About that time some wise men from eastern lands arrived in Jerusalem, asking, "Where is the newborn king of the Jews? We saw his star as it rose, and we have come to worship him."

King Herod was deeply disturbed when he heard this, as was everyone in Jerusalem. He called a meeting of the leading priests and asked, "Where is the Messiah supposed to be born?"

"In Bethlehem," they said,

Matthew 2:7–8
Then Herod called for a private meeting with the wise men, and he learned from them the time when the star first appeared. Then he told them, "Go to Bethlehem and search carefully for the child. And when you find him, come back and tell me so that I can go and worship him, too!"

Matthew 2:9, 11
After this interview the wise men went their way. And the star they had seen in the east guided them to Bethlehem. It went ahead of them and stopped over the place where the child was. They entered the house and saw the child with his mother, Mary, and they bowed down and worshiped him. Then they opened their treasure chests and gave him gifts of gold, frankincense, and myrrh.
*Gold was for a king, priests burned frankincense, and myrrh was used for the dead. Jesus is our king and high priest, and he died for you and me!

Matthew 2:12
When it was time to leave, they returned to their own country by another route, for God had warned them in a dream not to return to Herod.

Matthew 2:16
Herod was furious when he realized that the wise men had outwitted him. He sent soldiers to kill all the boys in and around Bethlehem who were two years old and under, based on the wise men's report of the star's first appearance.

*The fifth angelic visitation was:
Matthew 2:13-14  *The Escape to Egypt*

After the wise men were gone, an angel of the Lord appeared to Joseph in a dream. "Get up! Flee to Egypt with the child and his mother," the angel said. "Stay there until I tell you to return, because Herod is going to search for the child to kill him." That night Joseph left for Egypt with the child and Mary, his mother,
*Joseph must have arisen in the middle of the night and quietly left Bethlehem for Egypt.

*Since they received gifts from the wise men, they were well equipped to begin a new life in a foreign land. Jesus was around 18-24 months when they left Bethlehem.

Matthew 2:19–20  *The Return to Nazareth*
When Herod died, an angel of the Lord appeared in a dream to Joseph in Egypt. "Get up!" the angel said. "Take the child and his mother back to the land of Israel, because those who were trying to kill the child are dead."
*This was the sixth angelic visitation.

Matthew 2:21

So Joseph got up and returned to the land of Israel with Jesus and his mother.
*Jesus was three to four years old when they returned.

Matthew 2:22

But when he learned that the new ruler of Judea was Herod's son Archelaus, he was afraid to go there. Then, after being warned in a dream, he left for the region of Galilee.
*This was the seven angelic visitation surrounding the birth of Christ. This is the most angelic visitations recorded in such a short period in the Bible.

*Author's notes

## Chapter 24

# REVELATION OF THE MESSIAH THROUGH THE POWER OF THE HOLY SPIRIT

In this theme, we will explore who knew Jesus was the Messiah. I use this idea in December, the week after the angelic visitation theme. These two topics build upon each other to give us the whole story surrounding Jesus' birth in Luke and Matthew.

Luke 1:11, 13-15 (ESV)
And there appeared to him an angel of the Lord standing on the right side of the altar of incense. But the angel said to him, "Do not be afraid, Zechariah, for your prayer has been heard, and your wife Elizabeth will bear you a son, and you shall call his name John. And you will have joy and gladness, and many will rejoice at his birth, for he will be great before the Lord. And he must not drink wine or strong drink, and he will be filled with the Holy Spirit, even from his mother's womb."
*The child they speak of was John the Baptist.

Luke 1:26-27, 28a, 31–33
In the sixth month of Elizabeth's pregnancy, God sent the angel Gabriel to Nazareth, to a virgin named Mary. She was engaged to be married to a man named Joseph. Gabriel appeared to her and said, "You will conceive and give birth to a son, and you will name him Jesus. He will be very great and will be called the Son of the Most High. The Lord God

will give him the throne of his ancestor David. And he will reign over Israel forever; his Kingdom will never end!"

Luke 1:36
What's more, your relative Elizabeth has become pregnant in her old age! People used to say she was barren, but she has conceived a son and is now in her sixth month.

Luke 1:39–40 *Mary Visits Elizabeth*
A few days later Mary hurried to the hill country of Judea, to the town where Zechariah lived. She entered the house and greeted Elizabeth.
*Mary must have been escorted by a family member to where Elizabeth lived, near Jerusalem.

Luke 1:41–45 (ESV)
And when Elizabeth heard the greeting of Mary, the baby leaped in her womb. And Elizabeth was filled with the Holy Spirit, and she exclaimed with a loud cry, "Blessed are you among women, and blessed is the fruit of your womb! And why is this granted to me that the mother of my Lord should come to me? For behold, when the sound of your greeting came to my ears, the baby in my womb leaped for joy. And blessed is she who believed that there would be a fulfillment of what was spoken to her from the Lord."

*Mary stayed with Elizabeth for her last three months of pregnancy. She must have been a great help to Elizabeth, who was old.
Luke 1:57–64 *The Birth of John the Baptist*
When it was time for Elizabeth's baby to be born, she gave birth to a son. And when her neighbors and relatives heard that the Lord had been very merciful to her, everyone rejoiced with her.

When the baby was eight days old, they all came for the circumcision ceremony. They wanted to name him Zechariah, after his father. But Elizabeth said, "No! His name is John!"

"What?" they exclaimed. "There is no one in all your family by that name." So they used gestures to ask the baby's father what he wanted to name him. He motioned for a writing tablet, and to everyone's surprise he wrote, "His name is John." Instantly Zechariah could speak again, and he began praising God.

Luke 1:67, 76–77  *Zechariah's Prophecy*
Then his father, Zechariah, was filled with the Holy Spirit and gave this prophecy:
"And you, my little son, will be called the prophet of the Most High, because you will prepare the way for the Lord. You will tell his people how to find salvation through forgiveness of their sins."

*After John's birth, Mary came home to Nazareth, and it was apparent she was pregnant.
Matthew 1:18–21  *The Birth of Jesus the Messiah*
This is how Jesus the Messiah was born. His mother, Mary, was engaged to be married to Joseph. But before the marriage took place, while she was still a virgin, she became pregnant through the power of the Holy Spirit. Joseph, her fiancé, was a good man and did not want to disgrace her publicly, so he decided to break the engagement quietly.
As he considered this, an angel of the Lord appeared to him in a dream. "Joseph, son of David," the angel said, "do not be afraid to take Mary as your wife. For the child within her was conceived by the Holy Spirit. And she will have a son, and you are to name him Jesus, for he will save his people from their sins."

*If you look at the previous two Scripture you will find:
1. Zechariah prophesied that John would tell his people how to find salvation through the forgiveness of their sins.

2. Gabriel said Jesus would save his people from their sins.

*Now, I reiterate that Mary, Joseph, Elizabeth, and Zechariah knew the baby that Mary carried was the Messiah.

Luke 2:8, 10-12  *The Shepherds and Angels*
That night there were shepherds staying in the fields nearby, guarding their flocks of sheep.
but the angel reassured them. "Don't be afraid!" he said. "I bring you good news that will bring great joy to all people. The Savior—yes, the Messiah, the Lord—has been born today in Bethlehem, the city of David! And you will recognize him by this sign: You will find a baby wrapped snugly in strips of cloth, lying in a manger."

Luke 2:15–18
When the angels had returned to heaven, the shepherds said to each other, "Let's go to Bethlehem! Let's see this thing that has happened, which the Lord has told us about."
They hurried to the village and found Mary and Joseph. And there was the baby, lying in the manger. After seeing him, the shepherds told everyone what had happened and what the angel had said to them about this child. All who heard the shepherds' story were astonished,

*Now why do you think Mary and Joseph chose to stay in Bethlehem, where they were famed, versus going back to Nazareth where they were the center of gossip?

Luke 2:21-24a
Eight days later, when the baby was circumcised, he was named Jesus, the name given him by the angel even before he was conceived. Then it was time for their purification offering, as required by the law of Moses after the birth of a child; so his parents took him to Jerusalem to present him to the Lord. The law of the Lord says, "If a woman's first child is

a boy, he must be dedicated to the Lord." So they offered the sacrifice required in the law of the Lord.

## Luke 2:25–35  *The Prophecy of Simeon*

At that time there was a man in Jerusalem named Simeon. He was righteous and devout and was eagerly waiting for the Messiah to come and rescue Israel. The Holy Spirit was upon him and had revealed to him that he would not die until he had seen the Lord's Messiah. That day the Spirit led him to the Temple. So when Mary and Joseph came to present the baby Jesus to the Lord as the law required, Simeon was there. He took the child in his arms and praised God, saying,

"Sovereign Lord, now let your servant die in peace, as you have promised.

I have seen your salvation, which you have prepared for all people.

He is a light to reveal God to the nations, and he is the glory of your people Israel!"

Jesus' parents were amazed at what was being said about him. Then Simeon blessed them, and he said to Mary, the baby's mother, "This child is destined to cause many in Israel to fall, but he will be a joy to many others. He has been sent as a sign from God, but many will oppose him. As a result, the deepest thoughts of many hearts will be revealed. And a sword will pierce your very soul."

*The shepherds and Simeon knew that Jesus was the Messiah.

## Luke 2:19

but Mary kept all these things in her heart and thought about them often.

## Luke 2:52 (RSV)

And Jesus increased in wisdom and in stature, and in favor with God and man.

*Jesus began his ministry by being baptized by Elizabeth's son, John.
John 1:29–34 *Jesus, the Lamb of God*

The next day John saw Jesus coming toward him and said, "Look! The Lamb of God who takes away the sin of the world! He is the one I was talking about when I said, 'A man is coming after me who is far greater than I am, for he existed long before me.' I did not recognize him as the Messiah, but I have been baptizing with water so that he might be revealed to Israel."

Then John testified, "I saw the Holy Spirit descending like a dove from heaven and resting upon him. I didn't know he was the one, but when God sent me to baptize with water, he told me, 'The one on whom you see the Spirit descend and rest is the one who will baptize with the Holy Spirit.' I saw this happen to Jesus, so I testify that he is the Chosen One of God."

*Jesus asked his disciples:
Matthew 16:15–17

Then he asked them, "But who do you say I am?" Simon Peter answered, "You are the Messiah, the Son of the living God." Jesus replied, "You are blessed, Simon son of John, because my Father in heaven has revealed this to you. You did not learn this from any human being."

John 4:25–26

The woman said, "I know the Messiah is coming—the one who is called Christ. When he comes, he will explain everything to us." Then Jesus told her, "I AM the Messiah!"

*John, Peter, and the woman at the well knew that Jesus was the Messiah.

John 1:6-10

God sent a man, John the Baptist, to tell about the light so that everyone might believe because of his testimony. John himself was not the light; he was simply a witness to tell about the light. The one who is the true light, who gives light to everyone, was coming into the world. He came into the very world he created, but the world didn't recognize him.

Luke 18:8 (LB)
"When I, the Messiah, return, how many will I find who have faith (and are praying)?"

*Author's notes

*Chapter 25*

# THE LORD'S FESTIVALS

The information for this theme is from the book, *Celebrate the Feasts of the Lord* by William Francis (2012).

You may want to divide this theme into two yoga classes, as it is quite lengthy. I would cover festivals 1-4 in the first class and leave the last three festivals for a second class.

Leviticus 23:1–2  *The Appointed Festivals*
The LORD said to Moses, "Give the following instructions to the people of Israel. These are the LORD's appointed festivals, which you are to proclaim as official days for holy assembly."

*The seven appointed festivals of the Lord recorded in Leviticus 23 include:
1. The Passover
2. The Festival of Unleavened Bread
3. The Celebration of First Harvest or Fruits
4. The Festival of Weeks
5. The Festival of Trumpets
6. The Day of Atonement
7. The Festival of Tabernacles

*These seven festivals foretell Jesus' redemptive ministry on earth and of his second coming.

*Festival #1: Passover is celebrated on the anniversary of the Exodus of the Israelites from Egypt. Jesus died on the anniversary of Passover. Jesus was our sacrificial lamb.

*Festival #2: The Feast of Unleavened Bread begins the day after Passover. This feast is a reminder of when the Israelites fled Egypt.

John 6:35
Jesus replied, "I am the bread of life. Whoever comes to me will never be hungry again. Whoever believes in me will never be thirsty."

John 6:51
"I am the living bread that came down from heaven. Anyone who eats this bread will live forever; and this bread, which I will offer so the world may live, is my flesh."

*The unleavened bread of the New Covenant was the body of Jesus Christ, which lay broken in his tomb on the day of the Feast of Unleavened Bread.

John 6:32–33
Jesus said, "I tell you the truth, Moses didn't give you bread from heaven. My Father did. And now he offers you the true bread from heaven. The true bread of God is the one who comes down from heaven and gives life to the world."

*Festival #3: The Feast of First Harvest or Fruit was celebrated the day after the Sabbath right after Passover. The First Harvest was presented in the Temple as an offering to the Lord. This acknowledged Israel's total dependence on God.

*The year Jesus died the following events occurred:
Passover = Friday = Jesus Died

Unleavened Bread = Saturday = Jesus lay in the tomb
First Harvest = Sunday = Jesus rose from the grave
Jesus was our First Harvest

1 Corinthians 15:20–23
But in fact, Christ has been raised from the dead. He is the first of a great harvest of all who have died. So you see, just as death came into the world through a man, now the resurrection from the dead has begun through another man. Just as everyone dies because we all belong to Adam, everyone who belongs to Christ will be given new life. But there is an order to this resurrection: Christ was raised as the first of the harvest; then all who belong to Christ will be raised when he comes back.

*Festival #4: The Festival of Weeks or Pentecost was celebrated seven weeks and a day (50 days) after the Festival of the First Harvest. The Greek name for fiftieth was Pentecost.

*Ten days after Jesus ascended into heaven the following occurred:
Acts 2:1–3  *The Holy Spirit Comes*
On the day of Pentecost all the believers were meeting together in one place. Suddenly, there was a sound from heaven like the roaring of a mighty windstorm, and it filled the house where they were sitting. Then, what looked like flames or tongues of fire appeared and settled on each of them.

*During this Pentecost, the Holy Spirit descended and breathed transforming life into Jesus' followers (Francis, 2012).

*While Pentecost was a joyful celebration of Israel's grain harvest, it also commemorated the giving of the Law to Moses on Mount Sinai.

*The first four festivals given by God were fulfilled through Jesus' death, resurrection, and the dissension of the Holy Spirit. The next three festivals are yet to be fulfilled.

*Festival #5: The Feast of Trumpets or New Year's Day (for the Israelites) the Lord designated for the blowing of the shofar (ram's horn).

Isaiah 27:12–13
Yet the time will come when the LORD will gather them together like handpicked grain. One by one he will gather them. In that day the great trumpet will sound.

*This feast was a reminder that although the summer harvest season has ended, and the storehouses were full, each person must recognize their dependence on God.

*The New Testament pictures the trumpet as ushering in the Rapture.
1 Thessalonians 4:16–17
For the Lord himself will come down from heaven with a commanding shout, with the voice of the archangel, and with the trumpet call of God. First, the Christians who have died will rise from their graves. Then, together with them, we who are still alive and remain on the earth will be caught up in the clouds to meet the Lord in the air. Then we will be with the Lord forever.

*Festival #6: The Day of Atonement fell ten days after the Feast of Trumpets. This festival was a national fast day. On this day, the High Priest offered sacrifices for the sins of the nation of Israel to obtain atonement (reconciliation between God and his people).

*This Day of Atonement foreshadows the day of Israel's final repentance and reconciliation with God.

*Festival #7: Festival of Tabernacles
Leviticus 23:34 (NIV)
"Say to the Israelites: 'On the fifteenth day of the seventh month the LORD's Festival of Tabernacles begins, and it lasts for seven days.'"

*To commemorate the Exodus from Egypt, God instructed his people to live in temporary dwellings for seven days.

*The Festival of Tabernacles foreshadows the day when every nation will come to Jerusalem to celebrate during the Messiah's millennial reign.

*In summary: the seven appointed festivals included:
1. The Passover was the day Jesus died.
2. The Festival of Unleavened Bread was the day Jesus body lay in the tomb.
3. The Celebration of First Harvest or Fruits was the day Jesus rose from the grave.
4. The Festival of Weeks or Pentecost when the Holy Spirit descended upon the disciples.
5. The Festival of Trumpets will be the rapture.
6. The Day of Atonement foreshadows the day of Israel's final repentance and reconciliation with God.
7. The Festival of Tabernacles foreshadows the day when every nation will come to Jerusalem to celebrate during the Messiah's millennial reign.

*Author's notes

*Chapter 26*

# SCRUTINY OF YOGA

I do not know if you have experienced negative feedback from teaching Christian yoga, but I have. Two fellow Christians at my church went to the pastor and asked that Christian yoga not be allowed to be taught at our church. The pastor met with us and gave each of us an opportunity to present our case. Much of my platform from that meeting is included in this chapter. The pastor compared Christian yoga with drinking a glass of wine. If a person does not feel comfortable partaking in either (yoga or wine), then they shouldn't. However, that should not preclude the individual choice being made by each person. Ultimately, the class was allowed to continue and has since 2004.

Three months after this incident, one of the ladies apologized to me for condemning the Christian yoga class. She said God kept giving her the verse Acts 10:15 But the voice spoke again: "Do not call something unclean if God has made it clean." At first she did not understand what it meant, then God revealed to her that it was Christian yoga, and she should not condemn it.

Eventually, the second lady who opposed the Christian yoga class became an ally and assisted me in putting together a question and answer segment that is on my website: http://christianyoga.com. These are the pertinent questions:

**How is Scripture Yoga (Bible verses recited during the class) different from secular yoga?**

Scripture Yoga is different from secular yoga because you listen to God's Holy Word as it is recited in the yoga class. This allows you to be still and quiet while meditating on Scripture verses. The Bible instructs us to meditate on God's Word (Joshua 1:8). The Scripture Yoga class provides a worship experience while exercising the body he has given you develops inner stillness and quietness while meditating on God's Word. The postures for Scripture Yoga are the same as those used for Hatha Yoga. The difference primarily lies in the purpose and focus of the meditative session. Scripture Yoga is a Christ-centered approach that allows you to enjoy the physical benefits of yoga and experience communion with the Spirit of God.

## What is the history of modern day secular yoga? Is there any history of yoga related to Judaism or Christianity?

Stone seals with figures depicting yoga postures were found from the Indus Valley Civilization. This archeological evidence dates yoga back to about 3000 BC, which is before the beginning of Hinduism and Buddhism. This would be sometime after the flood and before the birth of Abraham. The term "yoga" was introduced around 1500 BC through the Hindu religion. Buddhism began its association with the use of physical postures and meditation around 600 BC. Therefore, yoga postures were performed by humans hundreds of years prior to Hinduism and Buddhism.

Interestingly, physical posturing such as bowing, lying face down, and meditation have also been associated with the Jewish and Christian faiths (Exodus 4:31, Psalms 1:2, and 143:5). Yoga posturing has not been associated with Christianity until the second half of the twentieth century. Christian meditation is foundationally focused on God and his Word, and this is the focus of Scripture Yoga.

The most popular type of yoga in the United States is Hatha Yoga in which the Eastern religion and philosophical portion of yoga are completely separated from the yoga class. In Hatha Yoga, the class is about performing the physical yoga postures and deep breathing. However, some secular yoga classes could still include portions of the Eastern religion. Therefore, if you are a Christian and want to do yoga, I recommend you perform Christian yoga. If you are in a secular yoga class, be discerning of the yoga teacher whom you are placing yourself under.

### If I like to do yoga, but I do not want to put myself in the environment of secular yoga, what alternatives are available?

Scripture Yoga allows the practice of posturing and meditation in a Christian context devoid of Eastern religious influence. In addition to Scripture Yoga (ChristianYoga.com), numerous Christian yoga classes are available on DVD (check out Amazon.com) or possibly taught in your city (Google it). A list of Christian yoga books and training facilities are listed in Chapter 27.

### Don't Hindus worship other gods while in these yoga postures? Am I worshipping a pagan god(s) if I put my body into these poses?

God knows our hearts. He knows whom we are worshipping when practicing Christian yoga and listening to his Word and thinking about him. God judges our hearts. Just as Jesus said in Mark 7:14–15, 20-23 Then Jesus called to the crowd to come and hear. "All of you listen," he said, "and try to understand. It's not what goes into your body that defiles you; you are defiled by what comes from your heart." And then he added, "It is what comes from inside that defiles you. For from within, out of a person's heart, come evil thoughts, sexual immorality, theft, murder, adultery, greed, wickedness, deceit, lustful desires, envy, slander, pride, and foolishness. All these vile things come from within; they are what defile you."

This principle can be applied to overeating, smoking, drinking alcohol, or being tattooed. These things do not necessarily defile someone. Exercising a certain way, including yoga posturing, is not wrong or sinful because God evaluates what is in a person's heart. Conversely, practicing Christian yoga outwardly doesn't make one right with God, although it does provide an avenue for God to impart his Word into your heart.

**My friends tell me yoga is dangerous, and I should not participate in it. To me, it just seems like exercise. Why are they concerned?**

Yoga is defined as "yoking" together. The exercises and stretches in yoga are designed to bring one to a place of meditation so you can yoke, or join with the spiritual realm. In Scripture Yoga, the goal is to prepare our bodies and minds to listen to the still, small voice of God. Some people believe participating in non-Christian yoga may unwittingly lead a person to yoke, or join to the spiritual realm in an undesirable way and expose them to dark spiritual forces (Ephesians 6:12). However, I have never felt exposure to evil spirits while in any type of secular yoga. In fact, Dr. Kevin Flynn, an Anglican priest, responded to this premise by saying, "Are baptized Christians, nourished by God's Word, one with God's people, really so susceptible to dark forces? I think not."

**Doesn't the practice of yoga within an Eastern religious context train your consciousness for a higher state of spirituality? Should I be afraid of that spiritual influence?**

Any practice, behavior, or form of worship that adversely affects your commitment or devotion to Christ should be avoided. We are called to be discerning and to test the spirits to determine if they are from the one true living God (1 John 4:1). The Bible says the body of a believer is the temple for the Holy Spirit, who lives within you (1 Corinthians

6:19). Scripture Yoga's focus is to lead you to the highest level of true spirituality, a relationship with Jesus. It should deepen the believer's walk with God by facilitating focus and concentration on his word as it is recited in the class. It provides an alternative method of exercise in a spiritually desirable and safe environment. Even so, Christian yoga may not be for everyone. As with all decisions, each person must choose for themselves.

I hope this book has been helpful in enabling you to focus your yoga class on Christ and God's Word. Now let me pray for you: Dear God, please allow this book to spread your Word, like seeds, into many hearts. May those seeds grow 100 times beyond what was sewn, and bless the sower, Amen!

Matthew 13:23

"The seed that fell on good soil represents those who truly hear and understand God's word and produce a harvest of thirty, sixty, or even a hundred times as much as had been planted!"

Sign up to be notified when a new deck of Scripture Yoga Cards become available at http://christianyoga.com/free and receive the free gift "The Fall of Lucifer." This is a brand new Scripture theme which is not included in this book. This Bible lessons answers the questions 'Why did Lucifer fall?' and 'Why do bad things happen?'

# Chapter 27

# CHRISTIAN YOGA TRAINING PROGRAMS AND BOOKS

I hope this book helped you prepare for each of your Christian yoga classes. It should impart much Godly wisdom to your participants. In addition, I have created Scripture Yoga Cards. Each card includes a yoga posture along with its corresponding description, and a Bible verse. Now you can grab your deck and off you go to teach! You can find the Scripture Yoga Cards at ChristianYoga.com.

Here are some Christian yoga resources. There are seven Christian yoga training programs in the United States. Here is information about each of them:

## Holy Yoga

Website: HolyYoga.net
Founder: Brooke Boon
Location: Moorehead, Minnesota
Certification: 95, 225, 500 hour Holy Yoga certification
Yoga School Established: 2006
Non-Profit Organization

## Living Waters Yoga/Yahweh Yoga

Website: LivingWatersYoga.com
Founders: Melissa Gray, Sarah Holder, and Marna Getz
Location: Lake Odessa, Michigan
Certification: 200 hour Yahweh Yoga certification

Yoga School Established: 2009
Registered with Yoga Alliance

## The Living Well Centers, LLC

Website: TheLivingWellCenters.com
Founder: Dawn Hopkins
Three Locations: Chandler, Arizona; Detroit, Michigan; Esterhazy, SK Canada
Certification: 200 hour Yoga Alliance certification and 300 hour Masters Certification
Yoga School Established: 2011
Registered with Yoga Alliance

## Lourdes Institute of Wholistic Studies

Website: LIWS.org
Founder: Barbara Moeller
Location: Camden, New Jersey
Certification: 200 and 300 hour Yoga Alliance certification
Yoga School Established: 1993
Registered with Yoga Alliance

## New Day Yoga

Website: NewDayYoga.com
Founder: Dayna Gelinas
Location: Kennesaw, Georgia
Certification Courses: 200 and 300 hour Yoga Teacher Training
Yoga School Established: 2006
Registered with Yoga Alliance

**Yahweh Yoga**

Website: YahwehYoga.com

Founders: Deanna Smothers and Courtney Chalfant

Location: Tempe and Chandler, Arizona

Certification Courses: 100, 200, 300, and 500 hour Yahweh Yoga certification

Yoga School Established: 2005

Registered with Yoga Alliance

**Yoga Faith**

Website: YogaFaith.org

Founder: Michelle Ann Thielen

Location: Based in Seattle, Washington; International School & Global Trainings

Certification Courses: 200, 300 and 500 hour Yoga Alliance Certification, Children's, Chair, Power, and other specialty certifications available

Yoga School Established: 2012

Registered with Yoga Alliance

The following Christian yoga books are available:

1. *Christian Yoga* (1961) by J. M. Dechanet OSB. He was a Benedictine monk.

2. *Prayer of Heart and Body: Meditation and Yoga as Christian Spiritual Practice* (2001) by Father Thomas Ryan, a Catholic priest. He also produced *Yoga Prayer* DVD.

3. *An Invitation to Christian Yoga* (2005) by Nancy Roth. It includes an instructional CD.

4. *Yoga for Christians: A Christ-Centered Approach to Physical and Spiritual Health through Yoga* (2006) by Susan Bordenkircher. It includes a DVD.

5. *Holy Yoga: Exercise for the Christian Body and Soul* (2007) by Brooke Boon. It includes a DVD.

6. *Christian Yoga: Restoration for Body and Soul - An Illustrated Guide to Self-Care* (2007) by Jennie Zach with DeAnna Smothers and Courtney Chalfant.

7. *Christian Yoga: A Daily Christian Meditation Guide for Your Practice* (2012) by Little Pearl and Julie Schoen (Kindle only).

8. *Stretching Your Faith: Practicing Postures of Prayer to Create Peace, Balance and Freedom* (2016) by Michelle Thielen, Founder of YogaFaith, includes three class, 90 minute DVD.

9. Scripture Yoga Cards: "Fruit of the Spirit" and "How to Receive God's Peace" (2016) by Susan Neal.


Other Resource:

ChristiansPracticingYoga.com website is an excellent network of fellow Christians practicing yoga.

# Notes

CHAPTER 2
Mark Water, *Scripture Memory Made Easy* (Peabody, Massachusetts: Hendrickson Publishers, 1999), 9-10.

CHAPTER 7
Beth Moore, *Loving Well Retreat in a Box* (Lifeway Christian Resource, 2005). This material was part of a retreat, not a published manuscript.

CHAPTER 8
Tim LaHaye, *The Spirit Controlled Temperament* (La Mesa, California: Tyndale House Publishers, 1994), 93, 95-97, 99-103, 105.

CHAPTER 9
Tim LaHaye, *The Spirit Controlled Temperament* (La Mesa, California: Tyndale House Publishers, 1994), 118-120,124,126,130,145.

CHAPTER 14
Beth Moore, *A Woman's Heart: God's Dwelling Place* (Nashville: Life Way Press, 1995), 210-211.

CHAPTER 21
Logos Bible Software 2004

CHAPTER 25
William Francis, *Celebrate the Feasts of the Lord* (Alexandria, Virginia: Crest Books, 2012), 6, 44, 46, 55-56, 67, 70, 77, 91.

# Yoga Posture Index

Chapter 4 contains the following yoga postures in this order.

1. Crossed Legged
2. Chin to Chest
3. Ear to Shoulder
4. Shoulder Shrug and Circles
5. Head Turns
6. Son Breath
7. Upper Body Stretching
8. Elbow to Knee
9. Seated Open-Angle Pose with Forward Bend
10. Seated Open-Angle Side Bend
11. Revolved Head-to-Knee Pose
12. Butterfly
13. Bent Knee Seated Forward Fold
14. Seated Forward Bend
15. Staff Pose
16. Seated Spinal Twist
17. Lion
18. Table
19. Cat and Dog Stretch
20. Thread the Needle
21. Cow Face
22. Pigeon
23. Downward Dog
24. Low Lunge
25. Camel
26. Yoga Mudra
27. Cleansing Breath
28. Squat
29. Standing Forward Bend
30. Standing Forward Bend with Leg Clasp and Halfway Lift
31. Mountain

32. Half Moon Side Bend
33. Standing Abdominal Lifts
34. Kegel
35. Warrior I
36. Warrior II
37. Standing Side Yoga Mudra
38. Posture Clasp
39. Triangle
40. Tree
41. Warrior III
42. Dancer
43. Eagle
44. Half Locust
45. Cobra
46. Plank
47. Locust
48. Bow
49. Child's Pose
50. Double Leg Raises
51. Boat
52. Reclining Spinal Twist (Two Knee Variation)
53. Supine Reach Through (Variation)
54. Bridge
55. Shoulder Stand
56. Fish
57. Wheel
58. Lying Spinal Twist (One Leg Variation)
59. Alternate Nostril Breath
60. Corpse Pose
61. Single Knee Hug
62. Knee Hug

# About the Author

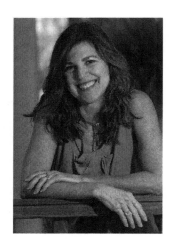

Susan Neal is a certified yoga instructor with over 30 years' experience in practicing and teaching yoga. As a pursuer of ultimate health, Susan Neal merged her practice of yoga with her spiritual practice of Christianity. Founder of Scripture Yoga, Susan recites theme based Scripture verses during her yoga classes. She produced two Christian yoga DVDs, *God's Mighty Angel's* and *What the Bible Says About Prayer* in 2006 and 2008 respectively. You can purchase these DVDs at http:// christianyoga.com. Susan published a second book, *Yoga for Beginners: 60 Basic Yoga Poses for Flexibility, Stress Relief, and Inner Peace* which is for the yoga student. Susan has also created Scripture Yoga Cards, "How to Receive God's Peace" and "Fruit of the Spirit." You can find her books and decks at: http://christianyoga. com/yoga-books-decks.

Susan teaches a free Scripture Yoga class every week at Woodbine United Methodist Church in Pace, Florida. She has been teaching this class since 2004. Additionally, she enjoys being a speaker and Christian yoga teacher at women's retreats. If you would like Susan to lead a Scripture Yoga class at your retreat, please contact her at SusanNeal@ Bellsouth.net.

Additionally, Susan produced a hospice CD, *Bedside Encouragement: When You Don't Know How to Say Goodbye,* which was designed to provide peace and comfort to those receiving hospice care. It would make an appropriate gift for someone who recently lost a loved one or has been diagnosed with a terminal illness. You can purchase this CD at HospiceCD.com.

You can follow Susan on:

https://www.instagram.com/scriptureyoga/

https://twitter.com/SusanNealYoga

https://www.pinterest.com/SusanNealYoga/

https://www.facebook.com/ScriptureYoga/

or her YouTube channel at https://www.youtube.com/c/SusanNealScriptureYoga

Please access the free Scripture Yoga class, "The Fall of Lucifer" at change the link to: http://christianyoga.com/free. This is a brand new theme which is not included in this book. This Bible lesson answers the questions, "Why did Lucifer fall?" and "Why do bad things happen in this world?"

If this book enhanced your yoga practice, would you please take a few minutes to add a book review on Amazon.com? Here is the link: https://www.amazon.com/dp/B01F5K8XQC. Book reviews are like gold to authors. Thank you!

Made in the USA
Middletown, DE
01 August 2017